Praise for
HEALTHY AT LAST

"I can personally attest to the truth Eric shares within the pages of *Healthy at Last*. This book exposes the injustices within our current food system and the evolution from slave food to soul food. It explains how what we eat is killing us and plaguing us with chronic illness, but not without offering a clear path forward toward eating to live and providing you with the tools necessary to take it. Eric's book will empower you to change your life and the lives of those around you."

— Rev. Al Sharpton

"Heart disease, type 2 diabetes, early-stage prostate cancer, hypertension, and other chronic diseases may often be reversed and prevented by changing diet and lifestyle. In this important and compelling book, Eric Adams describes how. Highly recommended."

— Dean Ornish, M.D., the father of lifestyle medicine and author of five *New York Times* bestsellers including *UnDo It*

"Eric Adams is living proof of the power that a plant-based diet has on the prevention, effective treatment, and even the reversal of type 2 diabetes. In *Healthy at Last* he delivers practical, life-changing, life-saving recipes for good health."

— Dexter W. Shurney, M.D., M.P.H., president of the American College of Lifestyle Medicine

"Eric's powerful story is so important and contains a message we all need to hear. *Healthy at Last* will motivate you and give you the tools you need to transform your relationship with food into one that is healing. I full-heartedly recommend this book. Never stop learning."

— **Papoose**, lyricist, entrepreneur, owner of Black Love clothing, and television star

"Healthy at Last furthered my appreciation of the power of plants and their ability to prevent and reverse chronic illnesses. The easy, healthy recipes included are *amazing*! Thank you, Eric, for this gift."

— **Remy Ma**, award-wining rapper

"To be healthy, we must educate ourselves on what's harming us and what's not harming us. *Healthy at Last* will educate and inspire you to take control of your health and change your life."

— **Fat Joe**, rapper and actor

"This book will inspire anyone who refuses to surrender to battling diabetes and high blood pressure. Eric is a true example that you can conquer disease with plant-based cooking."

— **June Ambrose**, creative director and author of *Effortless Style*

HEALTHY
AT LAST

HEALTHY
AT LAST

A Plant-Based Approach to
Preventing and Reversing
Diabetes and Other
Chronic Illnesses

ERIC ADAMS

HAY HOUSE, INC.
Carlsbad, California • New York City
London • Sydney • New Delhi

Published in the United States by: Hay House, Inc.: www.hayhouse.com®

Indexer: Joan Shapiro
Cover design: Jordon Wannemacher
Interior design: Nick C. Welch

Library of Congress Cataloging-in-Publication Data

Names: Adams, Eric, author.
Title: Healthy at last : a plant-based approach to preventing and reversing diabetes and other chronic illnesses / Eric Adams.
Description: 1st edition. | Carlsbad, California : Hay House, Inc., 2020. | Identifiers: LCCN 2020026112 | ISBN 9781401960568 (hardback) | ISBN 9781401960575 (ebook)
Subjects: LCSH: Diabetes—Popular works. | Diabetes—Diet therapy—Popular works. | Diabetes—Exercise therapy—Popular works. | African Americans—Health and hygiene. | African Americans—Diseases.
Classification: LCC RC662 .A32 2020 | DDC 616.4/62—dc23
LC record available at https://lccn.loc.gov/2020026112

Hardcover ISBN: 978-1-4019-6056-8
Audiobook ISBN: 978-1-4019-6073-5
E-book ISBN: 978-1-4019-6057-5

11 10 9 8 7 6 5 4 3 2
1st edition, October 2020

Printed in the United States of America

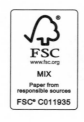

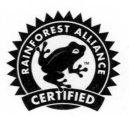

To my mother, Dorothy Adams.
You gave me the gift of life, and
then I gave you the gift of health.

CONTENTS

FOREWORD

I grew up in Chicago's South Side during the 1960s, a time when most of my friends and family ate what today we call "soul food." Think barbequed ribs, pickled pigs' feet, macaroni and cheese, fried chicken, and other foods that are deeply rooted in African American culture. These recipes have been passed down from generation to generation since slavery, and have been with us during the best and worst moments in our history. But the origins of soul food are more complicated: On the plantation, these foods were the scraps that white families refused to eat. Our ancestors were forced to make do with "food" like chitlins (pig intestines), ham hocks, and oxtail. It was up to ingenious Black slaves to find a way to survive.

I was fortunate enough to have a mother who came to see another problematic trait of soul food. When I was 11, she decided to enroll at the local junior college, where she took a biology class that would change our lives. Her professor had read about cholesterol and heart disease and their ties to diet. No one should be eating animal food, he explained, if they want to be healthy. My mom came home from class and announced that we were now vegetarians.

Thanks to that biology class, she learned what we all should have known: soul food is extremely harmful. And not just pork ribs and fried chicken, but all animal products. This is the source of so many African Americans developing premature heart disease, high blood pressure, diabetes, and other chronic diseases.

I embraced my mother's beliefs while learning the rudiments of cardiac pathology in medical school during the 1970s, and then cardiology training in the 1980s. As I discovered the innerworkings of the heart, I learned just how right my mother was all those years ago. Cooking and eating animals—especially in the unhealthy ways of the soul-food tradition—has helped African Americans become the sickest demographic in the country.

By the early 2000s there was extensive medical literature about both nutrition-induced mortality and about health-care inequities and poor outcomes in African Americans, but little about the intersection of the two. In the United States, Black people have a 21 percent higher rate of cardiovascular death compared to white people. That's due to several glaring underlying disparities: poorer access to care, lower levels of higher education and health literacy, and the implicit bias of some physicians and medical centers, to name just a few.

However, the usual diet of the African American community has become a nearly insurmountable burden on our health. Fried foods, refined grains, sweets, and animal products laden with saturated fat, cholesterol, and sodium all contribute to the pandemic of hypertension, diabetes, high cholesterol, and obesity, which in turn lead to heart attack, stroke, kidney failure, heart failure, and premature death. When combined with a lack of quality health care access, these underlying health problems also mean that African Americans are more than twice as likely to die from COVID-19 than white Americans.

After decades of diagnosing and treating heart disease, I've devoted much of my medical practice, leadership, and advocacy to helping people reverse their chronic diseases through plant-based nutrition. I'm proud to work alongside champions like Brooklyn Borough President Eric Adams, who wasn't as fortunate as I was to understand the dangers of animal products at an early age. He grew up eating soul food, and later, as a police officer, he ate its modern day incarnation: fast food. At the ripe old age of 56, he was diagnosed with type 2 diabetes.

His doctor said that his diabetes was permanent; he'd have to deal with the vision loss, nerve pain, and other debilitating effects for life. But Eric embraced the same plant-based philosophy that my mother did so many years ago. As you'll soon read, within months Eric was able to completely cure his diabetes and feel healthier than ever before. What's more, he was able to find easy and creative ways to honor our heritage by recreating traditional soul-food recipes with healthy plant-based alternatives.

In this wonderful book, Eric authoritatively intermingles history, nutrition, and the cultural practices that have had such profound consequences on the African American community. When he discusses "the chains that the Emancipation Proclamation failed to remove," producing the "Black package" of preventable, diet-induced diseases, I think of my own mother, who so wisely understood the dangers of unhealthy food long before most did.

As you read *Healthy at Last*, you might think that Eric's transformation is miraculous. You might think that his case is unique, and that you surely can't achieve the same results. But to me, his outcome was business as usual. I see it every single day in my office, with patients even sicker than he was.

And so, I want you to keep this in mind as you read: *You can do this, too.* If you have a loved one suffering from heart disease or diabetes, *they can do this, too.* Please join Eric and me on this plant-based journey. Together we can cure the health epidemic that has so thoroughly devastated our community—one bite at a time.

Kim Allan Williams, Sr., M.D., MACC, FAHA, MASNC, FESC
James B. Herrick Professor Chief, Division of Cardiology
Editor-in-Chief, *International Journal of Disease Reversal and Prevention*
Rush University Medical Center

INTRODUCTION

My Health Journey

In March 2016, life was good. I had the best job in the world: representing Brooklyn as borough president. I had just turned 56. I felt healthy. Maybe I was a bit overweight, but so were most people my age. I exercised regularly, and like all New Yorkers, I walked everywhere. I even got on the basketball court now and then.

I looked and felt fine—that is, until the day I woke up blind.

Terrified, I blinked my eyes rapidly, willing the world around me to come back into focus. Finally, I could barely make out the outline of my alarm clock. I stumbled to the mirror and saw, to my horror, that my right eye was bloodshot. I couldn't see anything out of the left. My stomach felt like I had swallowed acid. I had spent 22 years as a New York City police officer patrolling violent neighborhoods, investigating homicides, and raiding drug dens, but none of that prepared me for the fear I felt that March morning.

I immediately went to my doctor's office. The stomach pain turned out to be an ulcer, he explained, but my vision would probably be impaired for the rest of my life.

"Why?" I asked.

"Eric," he said grimly. "I ordered an A1c test, the one that measures your blood sugar percentage. A normal level is between 4 and 5.6 percent. An A1c level over 6.5 means you have full-blown diabetes."

"What's my A1c level?" I asked.

The doctor cleared his throat. "Seventeen percent."

Everything seemed to go numb. The kind of people who had A1c levels like that were wheelchair-bound and were taking regular insulin shots, or so I thought. I weighed 210 pounds—how could I be like them?

"Your high blood sugar damaged the blood vessels behind your eyes," my doctor continued. "That's what caused the vision loss."

"There must be some mistake . . ." I stammered.

He shook his head. "With that A1c level, you're lucky you're not in a coma." He whipped out his pad and prescribed insulin along with a battery of other medications. "Unfortunately diabetes is very common among African Americans, Eric. You're going to have to get used to the meds. You'll be on them for the rest of your life."

DNA OR DINNER?

All of a sudden, I had diabetes. It would define the rest of my life. Everywhere I went, everything I did, I would have to keep in mind: *Is this safe with my condition?*

At first I obeyed my doctor's orders. What else could I do? After all, he went through four years of medical school, a residency, a fellowship, and many years of practice to arrive at his conclusion. If he said I'd need meds for the rest of my life, surely he was right.

And so I went about my normal business. I learned to live with my impaired vision. But then came the side effects from the medication: the upset stomach and general fatigue. Moreover, the pills didn't help the general aches and pains I started having after 40. Whenever I saw a clock, I thought of my own life slowly winding down.

Like many Black people, diabetes runs in my family. We even have our own word for it: "sugar." When I was growing up, it seemed that everyone in the family eventually came down with it. After my aunt Mary was diagnosed with sugar, she brought a colorful pill organizer wherever she went. I thought that was normal. After my mother was diagnosed with sugar, she had to get regular insulin injections. That was normal. When my aunt Betty died of sugar at age 57—that, too, was normal.

I remember attending a family reunion with my mother not long after Betty's death. When we arrived, I realized Mom had forgotten her diabetes medication. "We have to go back for them," I told her. But Mom rolled her eyes and yelled out to the family, "Anyone have any diabetes medicine I can take?" Nearly everyone in the room pulled out a plastic case and shook their pillboxes in unison.

My family had pills that were every color of the rainbow: metformin, sulfonylureas, statins, blood pressure medications, and many others. As a kid I watched my family rely on these drugs, and now, at age 56, it was my turn. When I left the pharmacy after my diagnosis, I thought: *Is this really my future?* I had put myself through college, worked my way up from a beat cop to a captain to the New York State Senate and then to Brooklyn Borough Hall. I had a plan to become mayor of New York one day. I stared at those sad little pills in that sad little box and thought: *I've come too far to live out of a pillbox, man. There must be a better way. A healthier way.*

When I asked my doctor about other options, he held up his hands. "I'm sorry, Eric. There aren't any. If you lose some weight and stay on your meds, we might be able to keep your diabetes from getting worse. That's the best you can hope for."

That's the best I could hope for? I wasn't going to accept that. I wasn't going to accept a bad situation and just live with it. I certainly didn't do that after I was arrested for trespassing at age 15. It was a dumb thing to do, but the white cops thought it was appropriate to take me to the basement of the 103rd precinct, beat me up, and toss me into a juvenile detention center. Instead of accepting that this was how police officers would always treat young people of color, I vowed to join that same force and change it from within. As a police captain, I co-founded 100 Blacks in Law Enforcement Who Care, an advocacy group focused on improving relations between police officers and African Americans. When I was elected to the New York State Senate, I fought vehemently against the NYPD's stop-and-frisk policy and other forms of racial profiling.

There are some things you just don't accept, and bad health is one of them. My family and my doctor believed that sugar was genetic. It's just something that happens when you get older, they said, especially for Black folks. As a former police officer, though, I knew better than to take anything for granted. I was going to evaluate the situation based on the evidence and come to an informed conclusion, just like

I would at a crime scene. Was chronic disease and pain encoded into my DNA? Or was there something else going on?

The obvious place to look was my diet—one born from long hours on the beat. For many years I worked the midnight to 8 A.M. shift, so there weren't many quality food options available. There was only fast food. I became a connoisseur of the dollar menu. I'd roll my patrol car through the McDonald's drive-through at midnight for a double cheeseburger, swing by KFC at 2 A.M. for coffee and fried chicken, and throw back a few slices at Pizza Hut before dawn. If it was a particularly bad night, I'd hit up Wendy's for a shake and another burger and fries. For years and years, it was the same routine: fast, cheap, and easy meals—or comfort food, as you might know it.

For current and former police officers like me, comfort food means something deeper. It means safety. After responding to a multifatality traffic accident or to a murder, the last thing I wanted to think about was how healthy my food was. Picking up groceries at the store was not a priority. I needed food that would take the edge off. Psychologists have a term for what I experienced: *vicarious trauma*, also known as "compassion fatigue." While on duty I was calm and collected, but after, when I had time to process the horrors of the day, I relied on food as a coping mechanism. I self-medicated with Big Macs and milkshakes. French fries and chicken wings. Coca-Cola and nachos.

Comfort food helped me get through the aftermath of September 11. Hours after the Twin Towers crumbled, I arrived at Ground Zero to guard the search-and-rescue workers. We didn't know yet who had attacked us, and we were in constant fear. Nearly every restaurant downtown was closed except for one, an Italian place on Canal Street that stayed open 24/7 for first responders. We'd stumble in at 4 A.M., covered in toxic dust. The restaurant owner would shuffle out of the kitchen with plate after plate of baked ziti and chicken. Most of us were still shell-shocked from the attacks and shoveled the food down without thinking. We didn't care how many calories were in the buttered pasta, how much saturated fat was in the lamb, how much cholesterol in the salmon. Food was a respite, a constant, a support mechanism. Even later in my life, when I traded in my police sidearm for a suit and tie to serve in the New York State Senate, I depended on the same comfort food. If I had a bad day at the office, there was always a Quarter Pounder waiting for me. And there was no better destressor than passing around the KFC bucket with my family.

Ronald, Wendy, and the Colonel may have helped me get through some tough times, but they were taking their toll on my body. First the weight piled on, and then came the aches and pains—small ones, then big ones. My back hurt getting out of bed. My feet hurt walking to the subway. I was constantly tired. All of this became normal. Like all Americans who struggle with chronic pain, I soldiered through. I convinced myself that feeling unwell was just a natural by-product of aging. It was only a matter of time before I succumbed to the "Black package," as my family likes to call it: diabetes, high cholesterol, and high blood pressure. When I received my diabetes diagnosis, my mom was taking at least four pills per day: one pill to lower her blood sugar, another for her cholesterol, and two more for blood pressure. And at age 56, it was my turn.

But something wasn't adding up. Why was it that African Americans were nearly twice as likely to be diagnosed with type 2 diabetes compared to white people? I read a study in the *New England Journal of Medicine* that found that before age 50, African Americans' heart failure rate is 20 times higher than that of Caucasians. Was early death simply hardwired into Black DNA? Sifting through the data reminded me of the NYPD's "Heart Bill," which allows for special benefits and early retirement for officers who suffer from heart disease. The idea is that cops are *expected* to have a few heart attacks due to the stresses of the job.

Was I truly doomed to a short life because I happened to be a Black cop?

I wasn't convinced. After scouring the web, I came across research by Dr. Caldwell Esselstyn, Jr. of the Cleveland Clinic, one of the best hospitals in the country. Thirty years earlier, he had taken 21 patients with severe heart disease and put them on something called a whole-food, plant-based diet. I didn't know what that meant, so I googled it. Whole-plant foods are unprocessed and unrefined. Think of them as what you'd pluck off a vine or dig up in the ground. They don't have added chemicals to turn them into

Frankenstein foods, like potatoes into French fries or tomatoes into ketchup. They also don't have ingredients taken away, like brown rice into white rice. Finally, as part of this diet and just as important, you couldn't eat any animal products. No burgers, no fried chicken, no eggs, no dairy, no fish. I couldn't even use cooking oils. In short: nothing I could get off the dollar menu.

Food was more than sustenance for me. It was a part of my heritage. I could give up the fast food, sure, but what about soul food? I grew up eating my mom's cooking, and she learned the recipes from her mom, and her mom before her. The cuisine dated back hundreds of years, when my enslaved ancestors were fed the least desirable parts of animal carcasses, such as the ears, hooves, tails, and snouts. Slaves had to pioneer the use of spices and new ways of frying to make this food edible, and over the generations these dishes became soul-food staples. What would Mom say when I refused to eat her cooking? How would my friends react when I went to their dinner parties and asked for rice and beans instead of mac and cheese? The borough of Brooklyn is 35 percent Black. What kind of message would it send to my brothers and sisters—my constituents—if I gave up such an important part of our heritage?

I almost turned my computer off, but I had to know the answer: What happened to Dr. Esselstyn's 21 patients after they gave up the kind of food I ate every day? Nearly all of them reversed their heart disease and avoided any further heart attacks. Their arteries, once clogged with plaque, healed themselves after cutting out animal products and processed foods.

Could it be that simple? I dug deeper. I came across research by Dr. Neal Barnard of the Physicians Committee for Responsible Medicine (PCRM). His team took patients with type 2 diabetes and fed them nothing but whole-plant foods. Within weeks, "participants saw dramatic health improvements," Dr. Barnard reported. "They lost weight, insulin sensitivity improved, and HbA1c levels dropped. In some cases, you would never know they'd had the disease to begin with."[1]

You would never know they'd had the disease to begin with? The more I read, the more excited I became. I could get off insulin. I could get off all the meds. I could wake up energized and excited for my day— something I hadn't felt in many years. I could be healthy at last.

It wasn't just my own health I was excited for. My mother had been living with diabetes for more than a decade and was experiencing chronic pain. My sister was prediabetic. I was worried about my girlfriend, Tracey, who had been diagnosed with prediabetes. She is a public-school administrator who oversees schools in Brooklyn and the Bronx. I have never met anyone more devoted to her job than Tracey. She was so devoted, in fact, that she sacrificed her own health for the sake of New York's children. In addition to her prediabetes, she had had a hysterectomy for fibroids and was treated for anemia. At her most recent physical, her doctors warned her that A1c levels were on the rise. It wouldn't be long before she was as sick as me. I asked Tracey if she wanted to embark on this journey with me. We do everything together, and I wasn't ready to jump onboard unless she was.

"Let's do it," she said instantly.

Dr. Esselstyn generously agreed to speak with me on the phone, and he explained to me the science behind a whole-food, plant-based diet. He told me why meat, fish, eggs, dairy, and cooking oils had been slowly killing me for years, and how fruits, vegetables, whole grains, beans, nuts, seeds, and other whole-plant foods could reverse that damage and then some. "The human body is incredibly resilient," he said, "if only we allow it to be." I remained skeptical that I could ever enjoy eating this way, but I was determined to take charge of my health.

I replied, "Doctor, if this works for me, I'm going to encourage all my constituents to take control of their health just like I am now."

THE (SHORT) ROAD TO HEALTH

A few weeks later, Tracey and I boarded a plane for Cleveland. At the seminar, I was no longer borough president of Brooklyn. I was no longer a future mayoral candidate of the country's largest city. Rather, I was one of several hundred people who were suffering from chronic illness and desperate for a way to get healthy. I met people who had suffered three, four, five heart attacks and were wheeled around with oxygen tanks. There were folks who had been on insulin for decades and had terrible neuropathic pain in their hands and feet. Dr. Esselstyn's wonderful wife, Ann, prepared plant-based dishes for us to sample. Tracey, who was used to a steady diet of soul food and McDonald's, frowned and whispered to me, "What are we going to do, eat grass?"

I poked at the dark leafy greens with my fork, wishing that a bed of cheesy grits were hiding underneath. But then I tasted the vegetable biryani, the roasted cauliflower with tahini sauce, the sliced avocados, the quinoa cakes. It was incredible. Tracey and I finished our plates and stared at each other. This was not the sad, old rice and beans we were expecting. This wasn't the iceberg lettuce with tomatoes that we assumed vegans ate all the time. This wasn't rabbit food. This food was delicious—and, according to Dr. Esselstyn, could also reverse my diabetes.

"I want everyone here to give up one style of food that smells good, tastes good, and is absolutely going to destroy you and replace it with another style of food that looks delicious, tastes delicious, and is absolutely going to enhance your health," Dr. Esselstyn told us. The Big Macs, the fried chicken, the cheesy grits, and even Mom's soul food were destroying my body with inflammatory animal protein that wreaked havoc on what Dr. Esselstyn called our endothelium, the innermost layer of our arteries that acts as a life jacket for our blood vessels. The job of endothelial cells is to manufacture a protective molecule of gas called nitric oxide, which dilates our arteries and keeps blood flowing smoothly. But when we bite into that Chick-fil-A, that mac and cheese, that Whopper, inflammatory animal protein is stampeding through our blood and crippling endothelial cells, making our blood vessels stiff, lethargic, and prone to plaque buildup—the precursor to heart disease.

Dr. Esselstyn pointed out that many of us could have heart disease and not even know it. In fact, if we've grown up eating foods like chicken, beef, and cheese, it is practically guaranteed. Autopsies of accidental death victims in their teens and twenties routinely show arteries partially clogged with waxy plaque deposits. When you look at remote places of the world where people live mainly off fruits, vegetables, beans, and whole grains, western diseases like diabetes, arteriosclerosis (heart disease), and colon cancer are unheard of. In the now famous China Study, researchers studied hundreds of thousands of rural individuals living in China. In the Guizhou province, a region with some half a million people, not a single death over a three-year period could be attributed to heart disease among men under 65. Not a single one. Meanwhile, in the United States, 600,000 people die every year of heart disease. In my home state of New York, it kills 44,000.

"This," Dr. Esselstyn explained, "is the result of the standard American diet."

I looked down at my stomach. I thought about all those years sitting in my patrol car eating buckets of greasy chicken, beef, and pizza. Mountains of French fries. Ice cream sundaes. Each and every meal was poisoning my body. Like most American adults, I was likely already suffering from the early stages of heart disease.

My diet was also making my existing diabetes worse. I was one of 30 million Americans living with it, more than a tripling of cases since 1990, while Tracey was one of the 84 million living with prediabetes. As the disease progresses, it leads to kidney failure, vision loss, and in some cases, lower limb amputation. And for nearly 80,000 people each year, a disproportionate amount of whom are Black, the final symptom is death. I vaguely understood that type 2 diabetes occurs when the body builds up a dangerous amount of sugar, called glucose, in the blood. Normally, the pancreas pumps out a hormone called insulin, which helps shuttle glucose into our cells where it's used as energy. But people with diabetes like me develop insulin resistance, meaning the sugar lingers in our blood instead of powering our organs and muscles, which over time damages blood passageways and nerves. That's why I woke up blind one day, and why I suffered from nerve pain. That's why my mom required daily shots of insulin in an attempt to overcome the resistance.

Diabetics are almost always told by their doctors that their condition is permanent. They were just unlucky.

"With all due respect," Dr. Esselstyn explained, "these physicians are absolutely wrong."

He said that type 2 diabetes is a lifestyle disease; it doesn't happen unless we let it happen. When we gain weight from an unhealthy diet, fat builds up in our muscle cells, which blocks insulin from ferrying glucose to our cells. The problem is made worse when you eat a high-fat diet—that is, one with lots of meat and dairy. The fat from our food spills into our blood, further clogging up our muscle cells and preventing insulin from doing its job. Then Dr. Esselstyn told me that if I was able to remove fat from my body and animal fat from my food, I could reverse my diabetes entirely. Tracey could reverse her prediabetes. There was a possibility my 82-year-old mother could even reverse her diabetes.

It's true that some people might be more prone than others to developing heart disease and diabetes. There are some lucky people out there who eat nothing but Big Macs and sundaes and live forever, and there are people like me who get diabetes even though they're only a little overweight. But let me be clear: the scientific evidence overwhelmingly indicates that no matter your genetic predisposition, type 2 diabetes and heart disease can almost always be prevented—and in many cases reversed—by eating a healthy diet.

As I dove into the research, I realized that nearly every aspect of our health depended on food. I thought about my son, Jordan. Like most parents, I fed him meat, cheese, and eggs growing up. He drank whole milk every day. I followed the United States Department of Agriculture's (USDA) recommendations to a T. But when he was two years old, Jordan was diagnosed with asthma. To this day, he has to carry around an inhaler wherever he goes. I didn't know at the time that meat, eggs, and dairy especially have been found in studies to raise a child's risk of developing asthma. I didn't know that the antioxidants in fruits and vegetables could neutralize inflammation in air passageways and limit the asthma risk. I didn't know that even after his diagnosis, I could have reduced his symptoms by including large amounts of fresh fruit and veggies with every meal. Jordan may have gotten asthma no matter what, but didn't I owe it to him as a parent to do everything I could to make him healthy?

When Tracey and I got home, we took a long, hard look at our kitchen. The cookies, the frozen pizzas, the snack foods. Tray after tray of ground beef, pork chops, and chicken breasts. A small mountain of Big Mac cartons in the recycling bin. A greasy bucket of leftover KFC. We looked at each other and groaned. How had we been eating this junk for so long?

Tracey and I aren't people who do something halfway, so in one afternoon we tossed out every single unhealthy food in our kitchen. We tossed out all foods of animal origin. We tossed out processed snack foods. We tossed out sugary cereals and toaster pastries. Soft drinks and chocolate sandwich cookies. Beef jerky and cheese crackers. It was especially hard for Tracey, who emptied out food storage containers filled with her signature dishes. They were old favorites that made her think of her childhood, including the jambalaya with chicken that her mother used to make. The rice and hot smoked sausage recipe that's been in the family for generations. By the time the dust settled, we had emptied nearly the entire contents of our kitchen into a dozen garbage bags. Then we went shopping.

Immediately I noticed our first problem: finding quality food. After work I used to hit up the local bodegas for quick meals and snacks, but none of them carried fruit and vegetables. The closest thing to potatoes were potato chips. The closest thing to strawberries were fruit snacks. The closest thing to whole grains were corn flakes. Fortunately, in my area of Brooklyn, there were grocery stores nearby that stocked the kinds of foods that Dr. Esselstyn said I needed to eat, including fresh fruits, in-season vegetables, brown rice, and other whole-plant foods. On Saturdays I could get locally sourced produce from the farmers' market at Grand Army Plaza.

Except this wasn't the case for hundreds of thousands of my constituents. My friends in Brownsville, East New York, and other lower-income neighborhoods farther along the 2 train were less fortunate. They were served by bodegas, deli markets, and fast-food restaurants exclusively. How could someone eat a whole-food, plant-based diet in food swamps like this?

But before I could make Brooklyn healthier, I had to make myself healthier. I had to prove that eating plant foods could reverse my diabetes and restore the vitality that had long since left my body. I had to look and act the change I wanted to impart in Brooklyn. The first week was incredibly tough. It took all my willpower not to duck into McDonald's or KFC, or to hit up the food carts that were stationed next to Borough Hall. For years I had been their best customer. "Yo, Eric," they'd call out. "No hot dog today? No chicken and rice?"

"Not today," I'd say, jogging back to Borough Hall before I changed my mind. Instead it was a salad with black beans, tofu, tomatoes, and broccoli with tahini sauce back at my desk. When I was done with that, it was carrots and hummus. I snacked on edamame and trail mix. At 4 P.M., I had an apple and a banana. Whenever I was hungry, I simply ate more plants. Dr. Esselstyn assured me that eating plant based did not mean having to be hungry. Quite the contrary: I could eat as much food as I wanted and still lose weight and reverse my diabetes. It seemed too good to be true, but my stomach wasn't about to disagree with him.

At dinner, Tracey and I rediscovered our love of cooking. I couldn't make Mom's old soul-food dishes anymore, but I could reinvent them. We made vegan pot pie with cornbread crust using coconut milk. Vegan macaroni and cheese with almond milk and nutritional yeast. Oil-free sweet potato casserole. Vegan gumbo with beans and okra.

Almost immediately, the extra fat on my body seemed to melt away. After a week, I hitched my belt one hole tighter. After two weeks, my suit pants fit like a baggy parachute and my jacket sagged around the shoulders. People began to notice my dramatic weight loss. My deputy borough president, Ingrid Lewis-Martin, took me aside one day. We had known each other since the 1980s, back when her husband and I were in the police academy together.

"Eric," she said. "I'll be honest: you don't look so good. You know I love you like a brother, so be straight with me. Are you okay?"

"I'm doing very well," I replied, explaining that I had lost the weight on a plant-based diet. I had been harming my body for so long that everyone had become used to an overweight version of me. An unhealthy version of me. A diabetic version of me. But because I was losing so much weight, my body wasn't able to keep up. My skin was loose around my muscles. My eyes were sunken. And it didn't help that I looked like a kid playing dress-up in his dad's clothing. It was all temporary, and my body was still adjusting, but I *felt* healthier. I woke up with a spring in my step. I was no longer winded climbing the stairs of Borough Hall. I no longer felt exhausted by 3 P.M. Better yet, my vision cleared up entirely. Within two months of going plant based, I had shed 35 pounds.

When I returned to my original doctor, he looked at my new blood work and gasped. "Wow, Eric, I've never seen medication work this effectively before."

"I stopped taking my meds a month ago," I replied, grinning.

He stared at me. "I don't see how that's possible. Your A1c is below six. It's like you were never diabetic at all."

It was like I was never diabetic at all. Decades of poor health habits and tens of thousands of Big Macs, chicken wings, and French fries—all reversed in a matter of months.

Tracey was having similar results. She lost 30 pounds, and her A1c dropped so far that she was no longer prediabetic. Her cholesterol fell to normal levels. For years, she had suffered from exhaustion due to the stresses of her job. I thought being a cop for 20 years and running Brooklyn as borough president was hard, but that has nothing on what Tracey does. As a school administrator, she gets up at dawn to help run the largest school system in the United States. She never gets a break. Any doubts about eating plant based were put to rest when I'd see Tracey return from another 12-hour day still brimming with energy. Instead of collapsing on the couch, she'd asked, "What do you want to do tonight, Eric?"

Tracey and I were healthy at last. We had found a powerful tool and wielded it to heal our bodies. But something struck me as odd: *Why did no one know about this?* I had just reversed a disease that my doctor said was irreversible. And Dr. Esselstyn had cured dozens of people with end-stage heart disease. People who could barely walk. People who had suffered three, four, five heart attacks and were living on borrowed time. If it was that simple, that obvious, why wasn't everyone eating a plant-based diet?

SPREADING THE WORD

Meet my good friend Cliff. We worked together on the police force, and like me, he was a 9/11 first responder. He grew up in the Bronx and spent every chance he got on the basketball court.

He balled regularly until he was 52, when he broke his leg on a layup. After that, like so many middle-aged folks, everything else seemed to break down. Cliff woke up with constant pain from muscles and joints he didn't even know existed. He just assumed he was getting old. *That's what's supposed to happen,* he thought. Then, at age 58, came the prostate cancer—treatable through surgery, fortunately, but his recovery was long. Next came the hernia, which required yet another surgery and another painful recovery.

Cliff was an old man before he turned 60. One night, Cliff's heart began racing and he collapsed. He called his neighbor, who drove him to the hospital. The ER doctors told Cliff he had suffered a heart attack. He had a near 100 percent blockage in one artery and an 85 percent blockage in another. "If you had gone to bed that night," one doctor said, "you would not have woken up."

When Cliff told me what happened, I said, "Brother, you have to change up the food you eat! You need to cut out animal products and eat only whole-plant foods." I told him about Dr. Esselstyn's workshop in Cleveland and to check out the multitude of plant-based resources available online.

But was food Cliff's problem? Unlike me, Cliff ate a fairly decent diet for most of his life. He didn't eat meat or drink soda. He had a salad every day. But he devoured fish and dairy products. Cliff loved cheese, shellfish, lobster, crab, and shrimp. *Seafood is good for you,* he had always thought. That's what everyone was told. He didn't know that seafood is one of the highest sources of dietary cholesterol, that dairy is one of the highest sources of saturated fat—both major causes of heart disease. But after Cliff's heart attack, his doctor simply prescribed cholesterol-lowering pills. "Just take these and keep doing what you're doing," he said.

The former NYPD detective wasn't satisfied. "My friend Eric thinks I should try a plant-based diet," he told his cardiologist during a checkup. "He thinks all that fish and cheese might have caused my heart attack."

The doctor sighed. "That's probably too difficult for you. It's a lot of work changing your diet. The medication is a more realistic solution."

"What do you eat?" Cliff asked him.

He tried to change the subject, but Cliff pressed the point. Finally, the cardiologist replied, "The research suggests avoiding animal products can prevent heart disease, so, yes, I eat a whole-food, plant-based diet. Lots of fruits, vegetables, and nuts. And I don't use oil—that's also processed."

Cliff couldn't believe what he was hearing. His own doctor knew about the scientific research. He knew that eating animal products caused heart disease. But he didn't bother telling Cliff. Maybe he assumed that African Americans naturally developed heart disease as they got older, just like I had thought about my diabetes. Or maybe he thought that Black folks weren't capable of changing their diets and it was not worth giving them that information.

Cliff tossed out every last dairy product and fish stick. Every last block of cheese. The salads he thought had been healthy were actually ticking time bombs for his heart, thanks to the Thousand Island dressing and hard-boiled eggs. Gone was the sugar-packed yogurt he thought was part of a balanced breakfast. He tossed the cereals that had sustained him for years on the job. Within a year of upending his diet, Cliff had lost 30 pounds and dropped nearly all of his cholesterol-lowering medication.

Then there was my mom, Dorothy. She grew up in a rural town called Prattville, just outside of Montgomery, Alabama. Her family owned a small farm where they raised pigs, chickens, and cows and grew peppers and okra. Meat was on the table most nights of the week. In a time of horrendous segregation in one of the poorest places in the country, it was a big deal for a Black family to have steak and ham for dinner. It was a source of pride.

They ate traditional soul food, including buttered rolls with sugar, chitlins (pig intestines), pig ears, ribs, ham hocks, fried chicken, hush puppies (deep-fried cornmeal), oxtail, fried steak, and catfish. Some of these dishes might sound gross now, but they are staple recipes that my ancestors learned to cook as a means of survival, and they have been part of African American heritage ever since. Knowing what it was like to go hungry, Mom's family ate as much of the animal as they could. They seasoned the less-savory parts—the hooves, the intestines, the ears, the tails—in cayenne pepper, thyme, basil, sage, and other spices. When Mom moved up to New York in 1958, she got a job as a maid in Scarsdale, met my father, and moved to Queens. She got a job working at a day-care center, where she cooked for 200 school children. Mom still cooked the old soul-food recipes as she raised my five siblings and me, but fast food began taking over. Burger King Whoppers, McDonald's apple pies, Wendy's Baconators, and KFC Boneless Wings. She loved Little Debbie snack cakes. Fast food and processed snacks were cheap, convenient, and delicious.

Then came the health problems. She was diagnosed with diabetes in the mid-2000s. Her doctor prescribed her medication. "It's under control," he said, "but you'll always have it." Mom was told to avoid sugary food and carbs, but the doctor said nothing about meat and dairy. But diabetes wasn't the only problem. She had high blood pressure, so her doctor prescribed beta blockers. By the time she turned 80, Mom was taking 12 pills per day for a variety of conditions. She was old, she figured. This is just what happens.

I had to help her before it was too late. But she was skeptical, mainly because of my own transformation. Once, I walked into her house in Queens down another 10 pounds, my shirt too loose around my neck, the suit jacket sagging around where my gut used to be. "Eric, baby," she said. "What's wrong? You don't look well."

"I'm fine, Mom," I replied. "I just changed up my diet. Maybe you'd like to try it with me."

Mom was reluctant, but I couldn't let her get sicker. So I took matters into my own hands. Later that week, my friend and secretary, Gladys, came by the house to say hello. Little did Mom know that she had an ulterior motive. Gladys opened Mom's fridge and tossed out the unhealthy food and replaced it with fresh fruit and vegetables. When she realized what happened, Mom called me at work and let me have it.

"What am I going to eat, Eric? You've gone crazy!"

"I love you, Mom. I just want you to be on this earth a little longer. Please give the diet a try."

Mom eventually agreed, but she wasn't ready to go fully vegan; she still wanted to eat the occasional fish, and cutting all cheese wasn't going to happen. And she would sooner die than give up her oatmeal creme pies. But Mom agreed to let me cook for her. I sent over meals every day. I introduced her to kale, brown rice, and beans. I made her red curry with steamed vegetables. Steel-cut oatmeal with fresh fruit every morning for breakfast. Mom was eating foods that she had never heard of before, let alone cooked for herself, but she stuck with it.

And then something happened that everyone thought was impossible: Mom's diabetes improved. After two months, her doctor took her off insulin entirely after being on it for a decade. She went from a dozen pills per day to only a few. Moreover, the aches and pains she had assumed were a normal part of aging subsided. She no longer had to dread getting out of bed every morning. For years, Mom had suffered from arthritis and painful gout in her joints. By replacing the highly inflammatory animal protein with plant protein, she decreased the amount of uric acid in her blood, which in turn reduced her pain. Now in her 80s, Mom feels healthier than she has in years—and she isn't even fully plant based. "I'm happier now," she says. "I learned that I don't have to eat all that meat. I would feel bloated and uncomfortable. Going plant based is the best thing I've ever done for myself."

After I became healthy at last, I thought about the promise I made to Dr. Esselstyn. If it worked for me, I told him, I'd devote my life to helping my constituents get healthy too. Nobody deserves to live with poor health when there is a simple and scientifically backed way to prevent, and often reverse, chronic disease.

In my capacity as Brooklyn borough president, I'm fighting to help New Yorkers of all colors, creeds, genders, and sexual orientations turn their health around like my mother, like Cliff, and like me. I'm working with hospitals and clinics to encourage doctors to disclose to their patients' dietary options for heart disease, diabetes, and other chronic conditions. In January 2019, I was proud to help launch the Plant-Based Lifestyle Medicine Program in conjunction with NYC Health + Hospitals/Bellevue. The program is actively recruiting New Yorkers suffering from chronic conditions such as heart disease, diabetes, obesity, high cholesterol, and high blood pressure and improving their outcomes through healthful lifestyle changes—including, most importantly, eating a diet rich in fruits, vegetables, beans, and whole grains and absent of animal products and added sugars. We began with 200 patients, and the waiting list quickly swelled to more than 650. The demand was so overwhelming that we are fighting to expand the program to ensure every New Yorker striving to get healthy gets the help he or she needs.

The only thing more important than helping sick people get better is helping our children stay healthy for life. The onset of heart disease, diabetes, cancer, Alzheimer's, and countless other chronic diseases begins in childhood, many decades before the first symptoms are noticed. I knew it was crucial to instill healthy eating habits in the next generation of New Yorkers, and that's why I fought to institute meatless Mondays in all public city schools. In 2017, barely a year after I reversed my diabetes, I stood beside Mayor Bill de Blasio to announce that 15 schools in Brooklyn were adopting meatless Mondays. Less than 18 months later, the program spread to more than a million children at every school across the city.

Now, I know what you might be thinking: *Well, Eric, you mentioned your story, your mom, and some old friends. What about the people you don't hang out with every day?*

Don't worry, I got you. If you're like me, you appreciate hard science, not personal anecdotes. You need to be convinced that it wasn't dumb luck that reversed my diabetes but genuine scientific and nutritional principles backed by peer-reviewed research. Well, you're in luck. In Chapter 1, we're going to take a deep dive into the science behind plant-based eating and see exactly why fruits, vegetables, whole grains, beans, nuts, and other whole-plant foods are the key to a happy, healthy life. You'll see that my experience, as miraculous as it may seem, isn't special. It isn't something that's out of reach for you. Whether you are suffering from diabetes, heart disease, obesity, or other forms of chronic pain—or if you simply want to prevent them—then read on!

No matter if you are well versed in the power of plant-based eating or if you are as naïve as I was that fateful day in March 2016, this book can help you along the path to good health. It will also arm you with the confidence and knowledge to sit down with loved ones who may be unnecessarily suffering from chronic illness. All they need is a little push.

If you are a person of color, I want you to pay special attention to Chapter 2, where we look at the history of soul food in America. If you're anything like me, soul food has a special place in your heart. Maybe you cook the same recipes that your mother and grandmother taught you. Maybe you just love fried chicken, chitlins, and other soul-food staples. This food doesn't just taste good; it reminds you of friends and family and shared community. Yet this isn't the food our ancestors ate in Africa. It's derived from the scraps that the masters in the Big House allowed their slaves to eat. While brilliant African American chefs learned to turn barely edible dregs like hooves, tails, snouts, and intestines into delicious food, we are not honoring our history by continuing to eat them. We are only making ourselves sicker.

You might be thinking that giving up unhealthy foods and becoming more active is too difficult or that it's too late in life to try. Well, it's not that difficult, and it's never too late. You can proceed entirely at your own pace. You can start by giving up chicken and replacing it with seitan. Or replacing pork with tofu. Maybe it's just replacing cow's milk with soy milk and taking the stairs instead of the elevator. Or beginning your day with oatmeal and fruit instead of a bagel and cream cheese. How about riding your bike to work instead of the subway? In Chapter 3 I'll lay out the simple and easy steps that I took to reverse my diabetes and feel better than I have in decades. I'll even teach you how to shop for healthy food in places that don't offer a whole lot more than Fritos and beer.

Finally, in Chapter 4, you'll get more than 50 delicious recipes from some of the best plant-based chefs on the planet. Don't you worry—it's not just rice and beans and salad. You'll have wonderful soul-food-inspired dishes like sausage-kale pasta, roasted veggie lasagna, and chipotle mac 'n' cheese that would make grandma proud. Pudding, chocolate truffles, and peanut butter cookies that will make your mouth water. You'll see that eating plant based is fun, affordable, and delicious.

Trust me: if I can become healthy at last after suffering from diabetes so advanced that I woke up blind, so can you.

CHAPTER 1

THE SCIENCE
OF PLANT-BASED
NUTRITION

Think about the people in your life who are suffering from heart disease and diabetes, two of the most common and deadly conditions in the United States. According to the Centers for Disease Control and Prevention (CDC), heart disease kills nearly 650,000 Americans every year. That's one out of every four deaths.[1] Type 2 diabetes contributes to more than 250,000 deaths every year, and more than a quarter of all seniors live with it.[2]

You might have members of your family who have these conditions. You yourself might have one or both, and you're looking for something, *anything*, to help you get better. In this chapter, we're going to discuss these extremely common conditions in depth for two reasons: because they are almost 100 percent preventable, and, in many cases, 100 percent reversible.

Maybe you're lucky and you don't suffer from either heart disease or diabetes. Let me ask you this: Do you want to avoid breast or prostate cancer? How about colon cancer? Arthritis? Do you want to avoid Alzheimer's and other forms of dementia? Depression? How about clearing up that stubborn acne or eczema? Maybe just simple weight loss?

Perhaps the simpler question is: Do you want to live a long life while remaining as healthy as humanly possible? If so, a plant-based diet is for you.

HEART DISEASE

After reading the introduction, you might think that the miracle of a plant-based diet—and that's what it truly is, a miracle—is recent news. Think of all the lives we could have saved if we knew about this 10, 5, or even 1 year ago. Except that we have known. We've known for more than half a century, and one of the first guys to figure it out wasn't even a doctor. He was an inventor named Nathan Pritikin.

A little background: Before the 20th century, dying from a heart condition was not especially common. Most people lived on farms and spent their time planting and harvesting crops. If they were lucky, like my mom's family, they had meat a few times a week. Yet as Americans became more prosperous and moved into cities, they began eating more meat. New advances in mechanization turned farms into factories that pumped out cheap meat for the masses. By the 1950s, America had won two world wars and the economy was at an all-time high—and so was heart disease, moving from the fourth leading cause of death in 1900 to number one. It wasn't unheard of for a man to have three or four heart attacks before he turned 50. The typical treatment? A week of bedrest. And maybe take the elevator instead of the stairs.

One day in 1957, Pritikin's doctor gave him startling news: his cholesterol was over 300, and an electrocardiogram showed that blood flow in his heart was severely diminished. At the ripe old age of 41, he had end-stage heart disease. Avoid all exercise, his doctors said. Take a lot of naps. Enjoy the time you have left. Well, Pritikin was a smart fellow who held dozens of patents in photography and aeronautics, among other fields, and he wasn't ready to sail off into the sunset quite yet. He had been reading about how people who had cholesterol levels under 160 were effectively immune from heart attacks. What if he could bring his own cholesterol to that level?

Fat chance, his doctors said. Cholesterol is genetic. You're just unlucky.

Pritikin set out to prove them wrong. But first he had to change the food he ate, which was pretty awful, even by my standards: three eggs every morning, buttered steak for dinner, a pint of ice cream for dessert, and bowls of whipped cream. He gave it all up and modeled his new diet on rural Ugandans, a group of Africans who ate the original soul food. Instead of chitlins, fried fish, gumbo, and red drink, the Ugandans were eating plantains, sweet potatoes, corn, millet, pumpkins, tomatoes, and leafy greens. Pritikin saw this in a study published in the *International Journal of Epidemiology*. After reading the very first line—"In the African population of Uganda, coronary heart disease is almost nonexistent"[3]—Pritikin knew he had made the right choice. Soon he was able to run four miles a day, and within two years of changing his diet, his cholesterol plummeted to below 160.[4] An electrocardiogram found that the blockages in his heart had vanished. His heart disease was cured.

Meanwhile, Pritikin's friends and family were still dying from heart disease. By 1960, it was killing a third of all Americans of all races and classes. President Dwight Eisenhower suffered a major heart attack while golfing and a stroke later in his second term. (Ike was a bona fide lover of soul food: his favorite dish was reportedly pig knuckles.) Pritikin was determined to help others reverse their own health problems. Over the next two and a half decades, he funded study after study to prove that a plant-based diet could prevent not just heart disease but diabetes, arthritis, glaucoma, and certain cancers too.

One person who followed Pritikin's advice was Frances Greger, grandmother of my friend Dr. Michael Greger. In the late 1970s, she was diagnosed with terminal heart disease. Her doctors had crammed as many pipes into her heart as possible to bypass blockages, but nothing seemed to work. "Confined to a wheelchair with crushing chest pain, her doctors told her there was nothing else they could do," Dr. Greger later wrote about his grandmother. "Her life was over."[5]

Spending her final days at home, Frances tuned into a *60 Minutes* segment about Pritikin, who had just opened up a treatment center in California. Despite terrible angina (chest pain) and exhaustion that kept her in a wheelchair, she made the cross-country journey and arrived at the center, where Pritikin transitioned her to a plant-based diet. Within three weeks, Frances was not only out of her wheelchair, but walking 10 miles per day. As Dr. Greger later wrote, "My grandma was given her medical death sentence at age 65. Thanks to a healthy diet and lifestyle, she was able to enjoy another 31 years on this earth with her six grandchildren."[6] Inspired by his grandmother's transformation, Dr. Greger went to medical school; founded nutritionfacts.org, one of the most popular online resources for plant-based science; and wrote the bestseller *How Not to Die,* which helped a new generation of Americans (including me) learn about the power of plants.

You probably recognize this next fellow who managed to reverse his heart disease: President Bill Clinton. Back in the early 1990s, when Clinton was running for president, he was famous for ducking into McDonald's for a burger and fries. He continued eating fast food and jalapeño burgers after his presidency, even after undergoing quadruple bypass surgery in 2004. Then, in early 2010, he woke up exhausted and looking pale. At the hospital, Clinton underwent emergency surgery to have two stents inserted. He recovered, but no matter how much plumbing surgeons shoved into his body, he would continue to suffer from severe heart disease for the rest of his life. Or so his doctors said.

Not content to be at the mercy of medication and bypass surgeries, Clinton reached out to his friend Dr. Dean Ornish, who, like Dr. Esselstyn, was an early pioneer of reversing coronary heart disease through diet. Clinton's doctors had explained that his bypass surgeries and stent implants were "fairly normal" for a guy his age, but Dr. Ornish wasn't having any of it. "Yeah, it's normal," he wrote to the 42nd president, "because fools like you don't eat like you should."[7]

That was the wake-up call Clinton needed. Since then, he has removed most animal products from his diet. He begins his day with an almond milk smoothie blended with berries, eats greens and beans for lunch, and has quinoa or a veggie burger for dinner.

When he's hungry between meals, he feasts on nuts and seeds and hummus. He also walks two to three miles each day. Since he decided to take control of his health, Clinton has lost 24 pounds and reversed his heart disease. "I might not be around if I hadn't become a vegan," he said. "It's great."

Now here's a wake-up call for the Black community: according to the American Heart Association, "Sixty percent of African-American men and 57 percent of African-American women have some form of cardiovascular disease that includes heart disease and stroke." That's right, over half of Black adults have sick arteries, many of whom don't even know it until that first heart attack or stroke. In the United States, African Americans have the highest rates of heart disease compared to whites and Hispanics.[8] Many people think that heart disease is something that only men suffer from; in fact, since 1984, more women have died from it than men on an annual basis.[9]

As I tell my friends and constituents every single day: it's not our DNA that's responsible for these frightening statistics; it's our dinner. Heart disease is caused when small bumps, called plaques, form in our arteries, decreasing blood flow to the heart and weakening it over time. When a plaque ruptures, the resulting clot can completely block blood flow, causing a heart attack. When a blockage happens in the brain, it's called a stroke. The cause of plaque buildup is LDL cholesterol—you probably know it better as the "bad" cholesterol. The higher your LDL level, the higher your risk of heart attack and stroke.

And what worsens LDL cholesterol? Your diet. "There's no question that diet has a huge impact on heart disease,"[10] explains Dr. Walter Willett, professor of epidemiology and nutrition at the Harvard School of Public Health. As we saw with my friend Cliff in the Introduction, a diet rich in any combination of meat, dairy, and eggs can clog our arteries. With every bite, animal fats are causing the buildup of plaque. A child who eats this way develops fatty streaks in their arteries by age 10. By age 20, those streaks begin turning into plaque. By middle age, blood flow to the heart and brain can be dangerously diminished. You can feel fine one day and then find yourself in the back of an ambulance—or quite possibly a hearse—the next.

Changing your diet can stop heart disease in its tracks. Dr. Dean Ornish, for example, took patients with moderate to severe heart disease and placed them on a plant-based diet. Blood flow to the heart increased after just a month, and after a year, their once-clogged arteries had significantly reopened without drugs or surgery. This was the first clinical trial showing that heart disease could be reversed by changing diet and lifestyle—and, in fact, Dr. Ornish even found more reversal with the group after five years. The results are the same no matter what color skin you have. Take it from Dr. Baxter Montgomery, a cardiologist based in Houston, Texas. Living in the barbecue capital of the world, he knows a thing or two about soul food. Like many African Americans, he grew up on fried chicken and gumbo. But after spending years caring for his mother, who suffered a series of long hospitalizations, and after lowering his own LDL cholesterol from 138 to 70 with a plant-based diet, Dr. Montgomery decided to devote his life to helping others reverse their chronic disease. He founded the Montgomery Heart and Wellness Center in 2006 with the mission to prevent and reverse life-threatening illness.

One of his patients was an African American named Betsy. She had the classic Black package: congestive heart disease, type 2 diabetes, and high blood pressure. Betsy's husband wheeled her into the clinic in a wheelchair, tethered to an oxygen tank. She had been given a death sentence by her doctors. Dr. Montgomery was her last chance. He took one look at her laundry list of medications and said, "Do you have a blender?" She was so close to death that he instructed her to consume nothing but blended fruits and vegetables. "Come back in 10 days," he said. Betsy wasn't even sure she could *live* another 10 days, but she followed his orders.

Not only was she alive 10 days later, but she was off her oxygen. She didn't even need a wheelchair. She was an entirely new person.

Dr. Montgomery told me about another one of his patients, Mike, who lives closer to my neck of the woods. A native of Harlem, Mike was on the waiting list for a heart transplant—his prognosis was that bad. While lying in his hospital bed, Mike came across one of Dr. Montgomery's YouTube videos about disease reversal. Tired of waiting around for a new heart, Mike decided he ought to try fixing his own. He checked himself out of the hospital, flew down to Houston, and began an intensive detox with a 100 percent plant-based diet under Dr. Montgomery's care. Eight weeks later, Mike was walking 10 miles daily. His doctor took him off the heart transplant list. He no longer needed one.

Mike and Betsy's experiences are not unique. "Stories like this are completely normal," Dr. Montgomery explained. "I see it every day." Most important, it's never too late to make a heart-healthy decision. Dr. Caldwell Esselstyn, Jr., who helped me reverse my diabetes, treated an 87-year-old man with severe heart disease who refused bypass surgery. Instead he chose plants, and today, at nearly 100 years old, he's still going strong.

Don't become a statistic. Heart disease is preventable and, in many cases, reversible. Have you given your heart a checkup recently? If you're over 35, get your cholesterol levels measured every three years. Generally speaking, you want your total cholesterol level to be under 200 and your LDL cholesterol—the "bad" cholesterol—*under* 100 mg/dL. But don't stop there. You can potentially get your LDL cholesterol closer to 70 or under if you eat a purely plant-based diet, which is about as close as you can get to total immunity from heart disease.

That means giving up all meat, dairy, and eggs. That's hard for a lot of people, I know, so it's okay to start small. Check out the delicious heart-healthy recipes at the end of the book for some new twists on your old favorites. You've got this, and remember, every bite counts.

DIABETES

Meet Kathy. By the late 1990s, she had lived with type 2 diabetes for the better part of two decades. She didn't have health insurance, so her doctor did little more than prescribe pills and shoo her out the door. By the time she met Dr. Milton Mills at her church, Kathy was in rough shape. She was taking insulin twice a day along with powerful blood-sugar-lowering medication. Nonetheless, her blood sugar still sat at 300 mg/dL—triple the normal level. She suffered from obesity and leg cramping so terrible she couldn't walk more than a block at a time. When she woke up in the morning, she had to sit on her bed for 15 minutes just to focus her eyes, which never stopped throbbing. The pain was so overwhelming that she quit her job. Fortunately, Dr. Mills had experience in not just treating type 2 diabetes but reversing it altogether.

Kathy was one of the 5 million African Americans living with the disease. The pain was relentless. It defined her existence. When Dr. Mills approached her offering a new treatment, she expected another pill, another needle, anything but results. Instead, Dr. Mills prescribed fruits, vegetables, whole grains, nuts, seeds, and zero animal products. Desperate for even a little bit of relief, Kathy agreed.

The transformation was astounding. Twelve weeks later, Kathy was off every single one of her diabetes medications. She was entirely off her insulin. She was off two of her blood pressure medications. Over the following year, she lost more than 60 pounds "without even trying," according to Dr. Mills. The blockages in her legs cleared up, and the cramping that had robbed her mobility vanished. Kathy could walk many miles per day, and she returned to work an entirely new person.

When I learned about Kathy's story, I thought back to my own diabetes reversal. I thought about how I nearly surrendered to the myth that with age comes chronic disease and pain. I nearly surrendered to the idea that my eyesight would never get better. After my diagnosis, my ophthalmologist instructed me to turn in my driver's license. "You are no longer legally able to drive," she told me. It wasn't until I visited the Cleveland Clinic that I realized all I had to do was get out of my body's way. With the help of good food, it wanted to heal itself.

Here is how a plant-based diet can reverse what was previously thought of as an irreversible disease. Those with type 2 diabetes develop a resistance to insulin, a hormone tasked with ferrying energy in the form of glucose (sugar) into cells. Unable to enter your muscles, sugar builds up to dangerous levels in the blood, causing damage to blood vessels and nerves. So what causes insulin resistance in the first place? Fat—both the kind that collects in your tummy and thighs and the kind you eat. If insulin is the key that unlocks the front door to your cells, body fat is what gums up the padlock. The problem is made worse by the fat you eat—specifically, animal fat. When you take a bite of that Big Mac or fried chicken, your body absorbs fat into the bloodstream, further clogging up the insulin keyholes in your cells.

The kind of fat you find in plants, though, doesn't do the same kind of damage. We know this by studying tens of thousands of predominantly plant-based folks in California. No, they're not hippies living in San Francisco; they're Seventh-day Adventists. Many of them eat a strict diet that steers clear of meat while emphasizing fruits, vegetables, whole grains, nuts, and beans. Scientists have long been fascinated by Adventists because they live as much as 10 years longer on average compared to the typical Californian. The Adventist Health Study 2, conducted by researchers at Loma Linda University, followed some 89,000 Adventists for decades and found an obvious link between diet and diabetes: Those who ate a "flexitarian" diet—meaning mostly plants and some meat—cut their risk of diabetes by 28 percent compared to the average Joe. Vegetarians cut their risk by 61 percent, while vegans cut their risk by nearly 80 percent.[11] In other words, the less meat, dairy, and eggs you eat, the lower your risk of diabetes.

The culprit is not just any fat, but *saturated* fat, which is found in nearly all animal foods and many processed junk foods. In addition to raising your cholesterol, saturated fat wreaks havoc in your cells by causing inflammation and increasing insulin resistance. The more saturated fat you eat, the more gunk that gums up the insulin receptors in your cells. But guess what: the fats found in plants do the opposite. Monounsaturated fats and polyunsaturated fats, found in delicious foods like avocados, almonds, and sunflower seeds, actually improve insulin sensitivity. That's why the risk of diabetes among vegans is closer to zero.

The most common question I get from folks struggling with diabetes or prediabetes is the dreaded C word: carbohydrates. It's a common misconception that if you have insulin resistance, you can't eat carbs; the idea goes that because your body turns carbohydrates into glucose, they raise your blood sugar to dangerous levels. In fact, carbohydrates are the single most important source of energy for your body, and they can and should be safely consumed, even if you have diabetes. The key is to choose whole grains, such as brown rice, quinoa, and oatmeal, which are absorbed slowly and safely. As Dr. Neal Barnard of the Physicians Committee for Responsible Medicine (PCRM) explains, "In a 2003 study funded by the NIH, we determined that a plant-based diet controlled blood sugar three times more effectively than a traditional diabetes diet that limited calories and carbohydrates. Within weeks on a plant-based diet, participants saw dramatic health improvements."[12]

That's right; you don't have to starve yourself to get healthier. You can actually eat *more* food and still lose weight and improve your blood sugar. Here's a fun thought experiment: What do 10 ounces of broccoli, 11 ounces of strawberries, 1.25 pounds of tomatoes, and 0.9 ounces of full-fat cheddar cheese have in common? They all have the same number of calories. Anyone could eat a cube of cheese, but a pound of tomatoes? Good luck. Let's try another one: Which has more calories, a 14-ounce bag of potato chips or a 9-pound watermelon? The chips, and it's not even close. They have 2,100 calories compared to just 1,300 in the watermelon. If you're like me, you've probably scarfed down a family-size bag of chips once or twice before—hey, it happens. But I'd like to see the hotdog-eating champion of Coney Island inhale a nine-pound watermelon in one sitting.

The point is: plants fill you up fast, so you can lose all the weight you need, lower your blood sugar, and stop diabetes in its tracks. And don't worry, you can eat a lot more than broccoli and watermelon. There are more than 50 delicious recipes waiting for you later on in this book to give you a head start.

CANCER

You didn't think we were done after just heart disease and diabetes, did you? While heart disease is still the number one killer in the United States, cancer is projected to pass it sometime in the 2020s. Cancer counts among its victims the very rich and the very poor, Black people and white people, friends and family. While cancer is not quite as preventable through diet as heart disease and type 2 diabetes are, the latest science does suggest that food plays a big role.

Let's start with breast cancer, which kills about 42,000 American women each year. Another 3.5 million are currently living with it,[13] including my sister Fey. I was heartbroken to read this statistic: African American women under age 50 with breast cancer have double the mortality rate compared to white women.[14] While billions of dollars have rightfully been spent searching for a cure, we've paid less attention to preventing it in the first place.

The studies involving breast cancer and diet are very promising. The Women's Health Initiative, a 20-year study of nearly 49,000 women, found that a diet rich in fruits, vegetables, and whole grains could cut postmenopausal women's risk of dying from breast cancer by 21 percent.[15] "This is the first randomized, controlled trial to prove that a healthy diet can reduce the risk of death from breast cancer," explained the lead study author. Conversely, the UK Women's Cohort Study, which followed 35,000 women, found an *increase* in breast cancer risk among those who ate red and processed meats.[16]

There's a myth out there that soy—a common staple of a plant-based diet—can increase breast cancer risk. In fact, the opposite is true. As the Mayo Clinic explains, "Studies show that a lifelong diet rich in soy foods reduces the risk of breast cancer in women . . . Soy contains protein, isoflavones and fiber, all of which provide health benefits."[17] Even women who have breast cancer can benefit from eating more soy. After following tens of thousands of breast cancer patients, a study in the journal *Cancer* found that women with breast cancer who ate the most soy lived significantly longer.[18] That's great news for soul-food lovers; some of the best southern-inspired plant-based recipes feature delicious soy foods like tofu and edamame.

Men, too, see benefits from eating a plant-based diet to cut their cancer risk. My father died of prostate cancer a few years ago, so I know firsthand how terrible this disease is. Every year 191,000 men are diagnosed, and 33,000 die from it.[19] Black men, unfortunately, are 1.8 times more likely to develop prostate cancer compared to white men, and the mortality rate among Blacks is 2.2 times worse.[20] Fortunately, research shows that prostate cancer responds very well to a plant-based diet. In the mid-2000s, Dr. Dean Ornish recruited 93 men with early-stage, "watch-and-wait" prostate cancer. Half the group continued with their typical diet, while the other half adopted a plant-based diet rich in vegetables, fruit, legumes, and whole grains. By the end of the study, the first group's PSA markers—an indicator of prostate cancer growth—continued to worsen. But the group who adopted a plant-based diet saw their PSA markers *fall*, meaning their tumors shrank. The worst food for prostate cancer appears to be dairy, which boosts the cancer-promoting hormone IGF-1; large scale analyses have found that eating lots of dairy increases a man's total prostate cancer risk.[21] On the other hand, lab studies have shown that drinking nondairy almond milk might actually *suppress* the growth of prostate cancer cells.[22]

When I read these studies, I think about my dad and his battle with prostate cancer. If only he had known about the power of diet—if only *I* had known—he might still be here today.

When it comes to fighting all cancers, the color of your skin doesn't matter; the color of your food is what counts. As the PCRM explains, "The more naturally colorful your diet is, the more likely it is to have an abundance of cancer-fighting compounds. The pigments that give fruits and vegetables their bright colors—like beta-carotene in sweet potatoes or lycopene in tomatoes—help you fight cancer."[23] For the best anticancer diet, each day I like to eat all colors of the rainbow, so think delicious strawberries, orange peppers, bananas, kale, blueberries, and beets, to name just a few.

You have the power to greatly reduce your risk of the cancer scourge if you give your body the chance. The latest research suggests that as many as 42 percent of all cancers and 45 percent of all cancer deaths are the result of lifestyle choices, so folks of all races and genders can benefit from choosing their foods wisely.[24]

ALZHEIMER'S DISEASE AND DEMENTIA

If you've had a friend or family member suffer from Alzheimer's or other forms of dementia, you'll know why it's called the "long good-bye." Alzheimer's steals our memories one by one, eroding our independence and turning us into shells of our former selves. Alzheimer's takes an enormous financial toll on the country—about $277 billion per year,[25] not including the time and effort caregivers must sacrifice. It also takes an emotional toll as we have to watch once-vibrant lives slowly fade away before our eyes.

Alzheimer's is a complicated condition, but one thing is clear: diet is a major factor, not genetics. Take native Nigerians, for example, whose diet is much more plant based compared to what you see in America. Their rates of Alzheimer's are four times lower compared to African Americans living in Indianapolis.[26] Likewise, Japanese men living in America have a much higher rate of the disease compared to Japanese men living in Japan, who eat much less meat and dairy. Similar DNA, different diet. No matter where you look in the world, the conclusions stay the same: the more animals you eat, the higher your risk of dementia. Meanwhile, the lowest confirmed rates of Alzheimer's in the world are in rural India, where people eat mostly grains and vegetables.

Over here in the United States, studies show that folks who don't eat meat and fish cut their risk of dementia by 50 percent.[27] "The best diet for brain health is full of whole foods like greens, legumes, berries, and whole grains, and is very low in animal fats, saturated fats, and salt,"[28] explain neurologists Ayesha Sherzai, M.D. and Dean Sherzai, M.D., Ph.D., directors of the Alzheimer's Prevention Program at Loma Linda Medical Center. They're a husband and wife duo who are at the front lines of Alzheimer's research, having analyzed studies comprising hundreds of thousands of people. Their conclusion? Alzheimer's is 90 percent lifestyle related. We have the power to protect our brains, our memories, and our independence.

All the meat, dairy, eggs, and processed foods we eat are causing inflammation and plaque buildup, which starves the brain of oxygen by clogging delicate blood vessels. This damage takes place over decades, which means the food you eat in your twenties contributes to the cognitive decline you might experience half a century later. You might not be able to travel back in time, but you can do the next best thing by giving up animal products and junk food now. According to the Sherzais, "Our combined research is revealing that early signs of cognitive decline can be reversed."[29]

LOOKING AND FEELING GOOD!

Okay, enough about fatal diseases. Avoiding the gloom and doom isn't the only good part about eating plant based. You'll also look and feel mighty fine the more plants you eat.

Let's start with simply getting out of bed. Not a problem when you were a kid, right? But maybe these days you're getting a little too used to the aches and pains you associate with aging. And for some people, those aches and pains are a bit more serious, with arthritis being the leading cause of disability among seniors in the United States. But guess what? Arthritis and other joint conditions are treatable with a plant-based diet. Take it from the good people at the Arthritis Foundation, who recently touted a study in which "patients followed a vegan diet for three and a half months and experienced significant improvement in tender and swollen joints, pain, duration of morning stiffness and grip strength than the people in a control group who consumed an ordinary diet."[30]

Speaking of feeling better about your body, did you know that heart disease affects more than just your heart? When men have decreased blood flow, they have decreased blood flow *everywhere*. The good news? When you reverse your heart disease and diabetes, you also reverse erectile dysfunction (ED). A study of men with diabetes reported that the participants had a 10 percent lower risk of ED with every daily serving of fruits or vegetables.[31] If you don't believe me, take it from the Oscar-winning filmmaker James Cameron, who recently produced *The Game Changers*, a documentary about elite vegan athletes. Says Cameron, "I'd love to put Viagra out of business, just by spreading the word on plant-based eating!"[32]

And there's nothing wrong with feeling good on the outside as well as the inside. If you have stubborn acne, you're not alone. According to the American Academy of Dermatology, 50 million Americans, including millions of adults, are afflicted by it.[33] But if you do much traveling, you might notice that people in less developed places of the world have clearer skin. In one study, researchers studying 1,200 mainly plant-based communities in New Guinea and Paraguay could not diagnose a single pimple in over two years.[34] The culprit? Dairy. Milk-producing cows are typically milked while pregnant, resulting in hormones in dairy products that may trigger acne breakouts in humans. Studies also suggest that other skin conditions, such as eczema, are linked to dairy products as well.

Finally, a plant-based diet isn't just good for your physical health; it might help your mental health as well. Depression, of course, is a deeply complex condition that is best combated alongside a mental-health professional, but recent studies do suggest that diet plays a role. In one large-scale meta-analysis involving 21 studies from 10 countries, a mostly plant-based diet rich in fruits, vegetables, and whole grains with "low intakes of [some] animal foods was apparently associated with a decreased risk of depression. A dietary pattern characterized by a high consumption of red and/or processed meat, refined grains, sweets, high-fat dairy products, butter, potatoes and high-fat gravy, and low intakes of fruits and vegetables is associated with an increased risk of depression."[35] So sometimes it's best to ditch the comfort food and fight the blues with greens.

□ □ □

Have I convinced you yet? Believe it or not, the science in this chapter is only the tip of the iceberg. I encourage you to check out pcrm.org, nutritionfacts.org, and other online resources to learn about the countless ways a plant-based diet can improve your health.

Eric, you might be thinking, *if there is all this science out there, why haven't I known about this before? Why didn't my doctor tell me about this?* We'll get to that in the next chapter, but to answer that question also means asking another one: How did Americans come to eat such a bad diet? More specifically, how did African Americans, who tend to suffer from some of the highest rates of chronic disease, come to eat this way? We'll see why becoming healthy at last means finally letting go of a style of eating that dates back to a time when our enslaved ancestors saw soul food not as a delicacy, but as a means of survival.

CHAPTER 2

THE
REAL ORIGINS
OF SOUL FOOD

In late August 2019, there was a disturbance in the universe: The fast-food chain Popeyes had run out of its wildly popular fried chicken sandwich after debuting it just weeks earlier. It was the logical conclusion of a frenzied battle that pit neighbor against neighbor, friend against friend, brother against sister. Who had the better chicken: Popeyes or Chick-fil-A?

Everyone had an opinion, from NFL stars to Cardi B to Justin Bieber. Fights broke out—both on Twitter and in real life. It seemed everyone had taken a side on the great chicken sandwich war of 2019. It didn't take long for the brouhaha to get racially tinged. Judge Joe Brown and Janelle Monáe bemoaned that African Americans were more concerned with standing in line for fried chicken sandwiches than voting, harkening back to odious Jim Crow stereotypes. It was a jarring reminder about the complicated history of what we call soul food—a southern-style cuisine with roots in African and African American cultures.

Like a lot of Black folks, I grew up eating soul food. Fried chicken, collard greens, mac and cheese, ribs, fried fish, sweet potato pie, cornbread, black-eyed peas—every Black family had their own recipes passed down from generation to generation. Our enslaved ancestors invented it as a means of survival, and today it's a way to bring families together. We eat it and remember how much progress we have made, and how much more there is still left to do. And yet, as we'll see in this chapter, soul food is also deeply problematic. It's cuisine that we eat to honor our past, but it is simultaneously compromising our future.

We'll start by looking at the history of three soul-food staples: fried chicken, chitlins, and macaroni and cheese. Together, they help tell the story of how African Americans came to eat the way they do. Then we'll explore the transition from soul food to fast food and how corporations have continuously exploited the important role food plays in Black families. By understanding this history, we can understand why unhealthy food is so intertwined with the African American identity, how it's impeding our economic progress, and why it's so difficult to give up.

FRIED CHICKEN

Fried chicken has been a culinary staple in this country for at least 150 years, though it didn't always come in a bucket or between a bun. The pioneers were largely Black women who lived on plantations, where slaves were not allowed to keep livestock. Chickens were the exception, since they didn't take up much space. These scrawny yardbirds weren't the meatiest creatures out there, so enslaved cooks needed to be resourceful by breading the edible parts, seasoning them with paprika and other West African spices, and deep-frying them in palm oil. After being freed, many entrepreneurial Black women sold fried chicken in markets and train stations.

Fried chicken became an easy and cheap option for Blacks who were regularly barred from eating in Southern establishments. Without reliable refrigeration, fried chicken also traveled well in hot weather. Though the cuisine was popular among all Southerners, white and Black alike, it wasn't until *Birth of a Nation,* D.W. Griffith's profoundly racist 1915 movie about the founding of the Ku Klux Klan, that it was associated with vile stereotypes. In the film,

Black politicians were portrayed as lazy and crude do-nothings who spent their days eating fried chicken and harassing white women—a not-so-subtle message about the dangers of letting Blacks vote. This racist trope has lingered stubbornly ever since.

In the 1930s, fried chicken went mainstream when a man named Harland Sanders bleached his beard white, dressed up in a white suit and bolo tie—harkening back to the good old days before the Civil War—and sold his fried chicken at a Kentucky service station. "The Colonel" would later become an ardent supporter of Alabama Governor and notorious segregationist George Wallace, who famously declared, "Segregation now, segregation tomorrow, segregation forever." (Sanders was allegedly on the short list to be Wallace's running mate in the 1968 presidential election.) Nevertheless, fried chicken has remained an important part of Black culture. It symbolizes the effort and skill of a people who have found a way to persevere in the face of horrendous circumstances. I certainly have fond memories of sharing fried chicken at my church growing up or passing a bucket around with my family.

CHITLINS

Another soul-food staple, chitterlings—or chitlins, for short—are also a dish born from slavery. They're a cute name for a very un-cute food: pig intestines. There's no better way to describe them. My mom would cook them growing up, and my siblings and I didn't think twice about what we were eating. I remember watching Mom dump an onion into the pot, which blunted the strong odor you get from stewing pig guts. Afterward she would batter and boil them, then serve the chitlins with hot sauce. They taste vaguely rubbery and salty; we'd eat them like dumplings.

As you can probably imagine, chitlins are far from the most desirable part of the pig. On the plantation the best cuts of meat— the pork chops, the spareribs, the tenderloins—went to the slave owners. The remnants went to the slaves, including the snouts, the tails, and the guts. It was up to resourceful slave cooks to figure out a way to make these parts edible. As recounted by the scholar Adrian

Miller in his book *Soul Food: The Surprising Story of an American Cuisine One Plate at a Time,* one former slave explained that "When we killed hogs, the white folks got all the good parts, least they thought that, and we got the neck bones an' ears, an' snoots, an' tails, an' feet, an' the entrails; what they called the chitlings. The white folks didn't eat any of that stuff."[1]

MACARONI AND CHEESE

Not all soul food is pig guts and oxtails, of course. During Thanksgiving 2011, then Secretary of State Condoleeza Rice was interviewed on the *700 Club* TV show, hosted by the televangelist Pat Robertson. Rice bonded with the co-host, Kristi Watts, over their mutual love of macaroni and cheese. A befuddled Robertson later asked Watts, on air, "What is this 'mac and cheese'? Is that a Black thing?"

"It *is* a Black thing, Pat!"[2] Watts shot back.

Indeed, macaroni and cheese has a special place on the dinner plates of African American families, which might seem odd considering the dish originated in Italy during the Middle Ages. According to legend, Thomas Jefferson fell in love with macaroni and cheese while serving as the United States' minister to France in the mid 1780s, even going so far as to ship a macaroni-making machine back to his house in Philadelphia. Jefferson supposedly brought his enslaved Black cook, James Hemings—none other than the older brother of Sally Hemings, the slave who bore six of Jefferson's children—to France to learn how to cook the dish.[3] Macaroni and cheese became a trendy meal for the wealthiest American families throughout the 19th century, and slaves learned to prepare it for their masters.

After emancipation, countless Black families had nowhere to go. The South was a devastated and desolate place, its economy in tatters. Most former slaves couldn't read or write, they couldn't get jobs, and they were the victims of horrendous violence. African Americans slowly emigrated to northern cities, where they intermingled with Italian immigrants. Many had their first bite of macaroni and cheese, which was no longer just for the white slave-owning families in the Big House. The dish was cheap, easy to make, and essential for Blacks who, despite being free, remained at the bottom of the totem pole.[4] Men worked for paltry wages in backbreaking places like railroad yards, factories, and lumber mills, while women were cooks, maids, and child nurses. They couldn't afford to eat much else besides macaroni and cheese.

FAST FOOD WITH A SOUL

Simple soul-food dishes like fried chicken, chitlins, and mac and cheese have been at the center of the dinner table through the most difficult and the most triumphant times in our history. They were there during Jim Crow, separate but equal, Brown v. Board, Emmett Till, the freedom rides, and Selma. They were there when we celebrated our progress after Barack Obama's inauguration, and when we cursed our lack of progress after Ferguson, Trayvon Martin, Eric Garner, and George Floyd. People sometimes tell me, "Giving up soul food is like giving up my soul itself."

Soul food, of course, is a fairly recent term. During slavery, soul food was literally survival food; it wasn't until the 1960s, during the Civil Rights Movement, that African Americans began reclaiming their deserved place in American culinary history. That's because to most white folks, soul food was just southern food. Everyone liked fried food and mac and cheese, after all. As Bob Jeffries, author of the *Soul Food Cookbook,* explained in 1969, "While all soul food is Southern food, not all Southern food is soul. Soul-food cooking is an example of how really good Southern [African American] cooks cooked with what they had available to them."[5] It's unclear who invented the term "soul food," but it was popularized by Sylvia Woods, who in 1962 opened her restaurant, Sylvia's, just blocks from the Apollo Theater in Harlem, the epicenter of Black culture and creativity. The "Queen of Soul Food," as she became known, served delicious soul-food staples including hot cakes, fried chicken, and ribs at her Lenox Avenue location. She served celebrities from Quincy Jones to Diana Ross to Muhammad Ali to New York City mayors, helping to establish the enduring legacy of soul food in America.

Pig feet and chitlins may not be regular dishes anymore, but we've graduated to something just as bad. If you walk a few blocks past Sylvia's, you'll find a McDonald's, a Burger King, a Popeyes, and a Wendy's. In fact, if you go to any predominantly Black neighborhood in New York—or any city, for that matter—you'll likely find more fast-food chains than grocery stores. According to a US Department of Agriculture study, African Americans over the age of two get a full 20 percent of their calories from fast food—more than any other demographic.[6]

This isn't by chance. It's the result of a concerted, decades-long effort by major corporations to fuse Black heritage with fast food—in effect creating a new generation of soul food. As the historian Chin Jou details in her book, *Supersizing Urban America: How Inner Cities Got Fast Food with Government Help,* this campaign began back in the late 1960s, after riots broke out in the wake of Martin Luther King, Jr.'s assassination. In an effort to reverse urban blight, the Small Business Administration, under President Lyndon Johnson, lent money to businesses willing to open stores in inner cities. Among the most eager recipients of this cash were fast-food franchises.

In the 1980s and early 1990s, as hip-hop groups like N.W.A. exploded on the airwaves, fast-food restaurants eyed another opportunity. KFC, for example, began piping rap and R&B tunes into its inner-city restaurants and retooled its menu to include soul-food staples like collard greens and red beans. Employees were encouraged to wear kufi hats, dashikis, and other clothing evoking African heritage. "We started looking at our customer base and found an opportunity to align ourselves with the African American community," explained a spokesman for KFC at the time.[7] In recent years, chains have launched campaigns such as Pride 360 (KFC) and 365Black (McDonald's), which organize Black-pride festivals. Meanwhile, advertising has become explicitly geared toward children to hook them on fast food for life. As the *Washington Post* reported in 2014, one study found that "fast food chains in predominantly Black neighborhoods were more than 60 percent more likely to advertise to children than in predominantly white neighborhoods."[8] Fast-food chains also tend to buy up large advertising blocks on TV channels popular with Black audiences, such as BET.

Not all of this is bad, of course. It's encouraging to see Black culture embraced by corporate America after being ignored for most of our history. It wasn't that long ago when Black people would be refused service at restaurants. Now they are inviting us inside, playing our music, and serving our food. And the food is so cheap that a family can afford to eat there for breakfast, lunch, and dinner. What's not to like? For many people, fast-food restaurants offer a sense of community. When I was a police officer in the 1990s, my favorite spots knew me by name, what items I liked off the dollar menu, and how I liked my coffee. They provided sorely needed jobs in some of the most troubled neighborhoods in the city. In many ways the warmth and happiness of soul food had become synonymous with fast food.

Whether it's Grandma's home cooking or a McDonald's hot apple pie, there is no denying that food plays an important role in African American culture. Some of my happiest memories are catching up with old friends over a steaming pot of mac and cheese, or of my mom laying a plate of ribs on the table. The food was important, but it was the people we shared it with that truly mattered. *That* is the legacy of soul food. It's the spirit of a people who have endured despite systemic discrimination and violence, who could not use the same bathroom as a white person just a half-century ago, who to this day are regarded with suspicion by police officers for simply walking down the street.

The problem is that this food is quite literally killing us.

THE REAL WILLIE LYNCH LETTER

To understand the darker side of soul food, consider the "Willie Lynch letter." According to legend, Lynch was a slave owner from the British West Indies who traveled to Virginia in the early 1700s to teach colonial slave masters how to most effectively control their "property." Using techniques like physical and psychological torture, Lynch purportedly explained how to pit slaves against each other so they wouldn't unify and rebel against their masters, guaranteeing that the institution of slavery would endure for centuries. The Willie

Lynch letter is almost certainly a fabrication, but its meaning hits hard at the core of what it means to be a Black American: that even with our chains gone, we are still a lower class of citizens. We are still being prevented from reaching our full potential.

As I tell my Black constituents, soul food is the real Willie Lynch letter. Because of it, we suffer from some of the highest rates of heart disease, stroke, and diabetes not just in the United States but the entire world. We suffer from chronic disease early in life, which keeps us from being productive and passing on wealth to new generations. I think about my friend Ken Thompson, who was the Brooklyn District Attorney from 2014 until his death from colon cancer in October 2016. Ken was one of the brightest people I've ever known. In addition to being Brooklyn's first Black attorney general, he was a renowned federal prosecutor and litigator. He became attorney general just as tensions over police-related shootings were reaching a flash point. Ken established a groundbreaking policy of not prosecuting minor drug arrests, and he helped to overturn the convictions of people who had been wrongfully imprisoned. He was a progressive beacon, and his life was cut tragically short at age 50 by a disease that is 50 percent more likely to kill Black people than white people. In fact, according to the American Cancer Society, "African Americans have the highest death rate and shortest survival of any racial and ethnic group in the US for most cancers."[9]

Is it bad luck? Do Black people have to deal with the enduring consequences of systemic racism in addition to DNA that prevents us from staying healthy during our most productive years? The science tells another story: In South Africa, fewer than 5 in every 100,000 Black people develop colon cancer. In the United States, however, 50 to 60 Black people out of every 100,000 develop the disease.[10] As we saw in the previous chapter, it's not our DNA; it's our food.

The scraps that slave masters tossed aside to keep us barely alive still have a stranglehold on our future hundreds of years later. As for Ken Thompson, it pains me to think what else he could have accomplished had he only understood the importance of healthy eating. It pains me to think of how many other brilliant African American minds have been extinguished prematurely simply because they ate like their ancestors. How are we expected to close the massive wealth gap when we struggle to make it to work due to chronic pain? How are our children supposed to close the education gap when they have to quit school to take care of a parent sick with diabetes?

It's a cruel irony that the food that is supposed to bring Black people together is actually tearing us apart, one fatal diagnosis at a time.

Dr. Milton Mills, a critical care physician and a member of the board of directors at the Plant-Based Prevention of Disease Conference, doesn't mince words when it comes to the legacy of soul food. "The food slaves ate weren't leftovers," he told me. "It was actual garbage. These people were confined to slave labor camps. They were worked to death. They were treated like animals and they were fed like animals. It's significantly different than what their ancestors ate. Studies have shown that when someone eats a diet that is more consistent with the West African diet, they have lower rates of heart disease, cancer, and diabetes."

Dr. Mills is alluding to what I like to call the original soul-food diet—the food our forebears ate before they were shackled, tossed onto a ship, and forced to work themselves to death on a plantation. Real soul food originated not on the tobacco fields of the Deep South but on the rice fields of West Africa. Before the height of the Atlantic slave trade in the 1600s, Africans in what are now Nigeria, Ghana, Mali, and other West African countries subsisted mainly on fruits, vegetables, and starches. A typical meal would have been a stew made up of yams and other root vegetables, grains such as millet and rice, and plenty of spices.

Hundreds of years before millennials discovered you could turn it into chips, kale was a staple of African cuisine. Kale, collards, and other cabbages were first brought by European colonists to Africa sometime around the 16th century, where they quickly became key ingredients in stews and sauces. Collards are, of course, a soul-food favorite today, but usually as a side to meat dishes. In the 1930s, Black sharecroppers derided collards without pork as "motherless greens"—that's how important meat became in the southern Black diet.[11] When I was growing up, Black families often judged each other's economic progress by how big that chunk of meat on the table was. If those collards didn't have a mother, it meant you couldn't afford one. That kind of shame lingers even to this day. That's not the case in Ghana, where greens are at the center of the plate and carefully cooked using dozens of elaborate techniques. Like contemporary West African cooking, meat was a rare luxury and was enjoyed more as a garnish.

For some of our West African ancestors, their first experience with meat came on the slave ship. The voyage to North America lasted as long as three months, and ship captains had to calculate the bare minimum amount of food needed to keep slaves alive during the nightmarish journey. This meant poorly preserved meat that went bad almost immediately. Slaves often had to be force-fed a heinous concoction of beans and rotting meat, known as "slabber sauce." Many refused to eat it and perished.[12]

Nevertheless, we adopted a diet born from slavery and made it our own. This irony is not lost on Reverend Al Sharpton, who famously went from 300-plus pounds to a cool 130 after switching to a predominantly plant-based diet. I've known the good reverend since the early 1990s, when I co-founded 100 Blacks in Law Enforcement Who Care. For decades, he has brought politicians from Bill Clinton to Bernie Sanders to Sylvia's Restaurant in Harlem. He uses Sylvia's iconic soul food to help educate our leaders about issues facing the African American community, but he avoids eating it himself. When he brought Mayor Pete Buttigieg there in April 2019, the Democratic hopeful feasted on fried chicken, collards, and mac and cheese. Reverend Sharpton had toast. "Soul food is not what our forefathers set out to eat. It's what they had to eat," he explained. "Why would we fight for freedom and keep a slave diet?"

NINE MILES AND THIRTY YEARS

The unfortunate state of African American health has much to do with the way slavery changed our eating habits. Science has proven it. In a 2015 study, researchers from the University of Pittsburgh recruited 20 African Americans and 20 South Africans and asked them to switch diets for two weeks. The African Americans ate a predominantly plant-based diet, with lots of fiber-rich foods like vegetables and beans, while the South Africans ate a typical American diet, rich in meat and dairy. After two weeks, both groups received colonoscopies. "We were astounded by the gravity and the magnitude of the changes," explained the lead researcher. "In Africans, the diet changes produced microbiota that were cancerous. All this happened within two weeks and was quite astounding. The more we talk about diet, this will be important for all Americans, but most importantly African Americans."[13]

In just *two weeks,* the American diet was laying the groundwork for cancer. Imagine the effects from years of eating fast food and soul food. It doesn't take much imagination at all when you consider that Black people have the lowest cancer survival rate of any ethnic group in the United States.

Food like chitlins, fried chicken, mac and cheese—these are the chains that the Emancipation Proclamation failed to remove. By continuing to eat the food our slave ancestors ate, we are perpetuating a form of oppression that is keeping us in the hospital instead of the office. We may not be at the mercy of the Big House, but we are at the mercy of Big Pharma.

We are also at the mercy of a health-care system that fundamentally treats African Americans differently than white Americans. Why is it that a baby born in Cheswolde, a wealthy white enclave in northwestern Baltimore, can expect to live to 87, while just nine miles away in the predominantly Black neighborhood of Clifton-Berea, a baby can expect to live to 67? And as *The Atlantic* reported recently, "In Chicago, a white resident in Streeterville can expect to live until 90, while a Black resident nine miles south in Englewood can expect to live until 60."[14]

What a difference nine miles makes.

Diet is a big part of the problem, but a lot has to do with fundamental differences in how white people and Black people are treated in the doctor's office. The *New York Times* reported that "A 2016 survey of 222 white medical students and residents published in *The Proceedings of the National Academy of Sciences* showed that half of them endorsed at least one myth about physiological differences between Black people and white people, including that Black people's nerve endings are less sensitive than white people's. When asked to imagine how much pain white or Black patients experienced in hypothetical situations, the medical students and residents insisted that Black people felt less pain."[15] A majority also believed a two-century-old myth that Black skin is thicker than white skin.

I don't mean to put down doctors. They are well-meaning and want the same health outcomes for all their patients, regardless of race. But this sort of internalized racism means that Black patients too often are not given the same care and attention that white patients are. Think about my friend from the police force, Cliff, who wasn't told about dietary strategies for treating his heart disease because his doctor didn't believe he was capable of changing his diet. All told, studies routinely show that African Americans are much less likely to trust their physicians and therefore less likely to seek out or comply with treatment.[16]

It's a self-defeating cycle, and it means that Black folks are getting sick sooner and dying earlier than everyone else in America. And the health-care system isn't doing anything to stop it.

The good news is, as we saw in the previous chapter and as my own experience shows, it's never too late to change your diet. The body has a remarkable ability to heal itself if we give it a chance. We can reverse the years and decades of destruction caused by unhealthy food. I see it happening every day.

Just ask Dr. Michelle McMacken, director of the Bellevue Hospital Weight Management Clinic in New York City. She helps countless African American patients cure diseases they thought were incurable. "Seeing someone reverse their chronic disease is quite literally one of the most rewarding things I have ever seen," she told me. While the fastest path to good health is adopting a whole-food, plant-based diet from day one, Dr. McMacken's patients see big results from transitioning at their own pace. "People have success starting with one plant-based meal per day. If you have chicken with lunch and dinner, how about we start by changing dinner to lentils, tofu, or tempeh? For other meals, how about adding in more vegetables so they cover half the plate? I always try to focus on what you're adding in rather than what you're taking away."

Do you think it's too hard to go plant based if you've been eating southern food all your life? Dr. Judy Brangman doesn't think so.

She's a physician in Raleigh, North Carolina, so she knows a thing or two about soul food. Even for her patients who have diabetes and can't go fully plant based, simple dietary changes go a long way. "Just by going 50 or 60 percent plant based, my diabetics have been able to bring their A1c from 10 or 12 to 6 or 7 in a matter of months," she said. "Everybody has to decide what they want to do and what changes they're willing to make."

So here's my question for you: What changes are you willing to make? How far are you willing to go to take control of your health? I'm not going to offer you an "eat this, not that" diet plan. You will stay in the driver's seat. If you eat plant based at home but sneak a few wings at a Super Bowl party, I'm not going to send the vegan mafia after you. You can even have Grandma's chitlins now and then if you really want to, though maybe one day you'll find some healthier plant-based ingredients to use instead. You can go plant based at your own pace. In the next section, I'll share my guide to becoming healthy at last. You might love some of my tips; you might hate some of them. Make an appointment with my office and you can tell me all about your experiences. No one does it perfectly, and no one has to.

Here's a secret about eating plant based: You can still honor your heritage and give up fried fish. You can honor Mama and Grandma and eat tofu. You can make meat-free crab cakes, crispy seitan chicken legs, mac and chickpea-cheese with nutritional yeast, biscuits, and vegan gravy. You can make Granddad's corn muffins with ground flaxseeds instead of eggs. Jambalaya with tempeh instead of sausage.

Remember, you can honor the best parts of soul food while throwing away the worst parts. You can honor our ancestors without eating what they were forced to eat. We are honoring their sacrifice by returning to our roots and reimagining soul food the way it was always meant to be: plant based.

CHAPTER 3

ERIC'S GUIDE TO BECOMING HEALTHY AT LAST

To help people become healthy at last, I am offering a simple guide based on the steps I took to reach my weight-loss and diabetes-reversal goals. These steps are straightforward, easy, and collectively can change your life.

I don't expect that you will accomplish every single step—at least, certainly, not by tomorrow. What I want to make clear is that becoming healthy isn't one large decision; it's an accumulation of many small decisions you make day in and day out, from skipping the coffee creamer to taking the stairs instead of the elevator.

I don't want you to think about the enormity of this goal. Instead, I want you to think about the first step you're taking by reading this book. You begin with one single step. Then you take another. Then try another one, two, or four weeks later. Maybe you'll get excited and try another 10 next week. Too many diet and health books require readers to follow a stringent plan that is so overwhelming, it's easy to fail. Not here. You'll follow the steps you can fit into your life, and maybe, someday, you'll integrate some more.

I want you to get healthier at your own pace, on your own schedule.

Before we begin, I will say that there is one step I need you to adhere to from the beginning: eating a mostly plant-based diet, preferably consisting of whole foods. Without this step, you won't see real change. You can bend the rules now and then, but a consistent whole-food, plant-based diet is the cornerstone of good health. Without it, all these other steps won't get you where you want to go. Without it, your plan to prevent and reverse chronic disease will fall short.

For some people, these steps will be easy. For others, they'll be more difficult. It doesn't matter. Short process, long process—it's all the same. You are constantly learning new ways to improve your health. You are constantly on the lookout for better foods, better exercise, and a better life. Good health is not something you have completed—and boom!—now it's over. Good health is something you have to work at all the time.

Start these steps today, and I promise you a better tomorrow.

GETTING
STARTED

CREATE A NETWORK OF SUPPORT

You, and only you, are responsible for your health. But it sure helps to have your friends, your family, and even your social-media contacts on your side.

Here's why: Certain foods can be highly addictive—especially the ones that are not good for you, such as sugar or dairy. If you've been spending your life stuffing your mouth with cakes and pies and cheeseburgers and milkshakes, you are going to have to get past your cravings for salty and fatty foods and develop a healthy diet. (Spoiler alert: once you are there, you will never want those foods again.)

Whenever you are trying to get over any form of addiction, you need support. Let your family and friends, and anyone else in your circles, know what you are doing. Have a serious conversation with them. Explain that you are concerned about your health, that you are going to try to reverse your ailments, and above all, that you need their support. This can mean anything from simply being there for you to making sure that they don't push you in the wrong direction by offering unhealthy foods—just as they wouldn't push an alcoholic in the wrong direction by offering up a drink. It's amazing how many times I've told people about my diet, and they've said things like "One brownie isn't going to put you in the hospital" or "One little hot dog won't hurt you." Well, maybe that brownie or hot dog won't actually hurt me, but it won't help me either, and it won't send me further down the path of good health.

Your family and friends should acknowledge that you need their help, so request that they be as supportive as possible. I have found that to be one of the most important aspects of this journey: the support members of your team. But some in the African American community may need an extra dose of help. Sometimes it seems that if you want people to dislike you, just tell them you don't eat the foods they love, like meat or cheese or milk. It can feel like you aren't just attacking their food; you are attacking their very culture.

I don't know of any cultures outside the African American community that have given the food they eat such a powerful, self-identifying name: we call it soul food, and we identify our food as something authentically Black. Your family and friends have to know that when you say you don't want to eat these foods, you aren't insulting the family. You're not insulting your heritage; you're not insulting your community. Just the opposite: you are trying to free yourself and your loved ones from bad food. When you say no to the food, you are not saying no to their love. You are saying "I love you, so I want us all to eat healthier."

Change your family's definition of love. Eat right.

That's why the African American community needs some extra support. When we finally eat healthy, we are not just freeing ourselves from a bad dinner; we are freeing ourselves from the diet our slave masters gave to us hundreds of years ago.

In addition to supportive friends and family, you need a supportive health professional. As you start off on your medical journey, your doctor will travel along with you as you progress to health.

What makes a good doctor? For one, it's someone who believes in the reversal of diseases like heart disease and diabetes. Strangely, not all doctors do. Many of you are familiar with physicians who will tell you that if you currently have a disease, you will have it forever. It has to be "managed." Not all diseases are reversible, of course. But the truth is that many can be reversed through dietary changes alone—that is, if you have the right information.

Next, does your medical partner believe that you must take medicine for the rest of your life for conditions like high cholesterol, high blood pressure, and diabetes? If so, then you might consider talking to another physician. (Or ask that your physician look at the research in support of your journey.) As we now know, pharmaceuticals are not the answer to many health issues. There are times when drugs are necessary. But far too often, doctors prescribe far too many drugs for conditions that can be cured by nonpharmaceutical steps, which leads me to the next question:

Does your doctor believe that a plant-based diet is better than an animal-based one? If the answer is no, then your doctor isn't aware of the latest research that we talked about earlier—the work that doctors like Caldwell Esselstyn, Dean Ornish, and Michael Greger have tirelessly reported.

Does your doctor believe that heart disease, diabetes, and cancer are solely hereditary? They're not. Genes certainly play an important role in our health, but with new research every year, the science of epigenetics is showing us that our genes are not immutable; in fact, they are far more malleable than we once believed. Through intelligent lifestyle changes, such as eating a plant-based diet, we can help forge our own genetic destiny.

How do you find such a doctor? I found mine by finding out who I *didn't* want. Once I learned about all the items mentioned above, I interviewed doctors recommended by friends and rejected them one by one until I finally discovered a physician who was open-minded, who knew about the benefits of a plant-based diet, and who was willing to help me along my journey to health.

Everyone needs a good partner who is part of their wellness team. Because that is indeed what you are doing: building a wellness team. Wellness is a team sport, not an individual one. Doctors are an important piece of the team, but they are not the entire team, and they must play their position.

No team member is more important than the others, so make sure that as you start your path to health, you find the right medical practitioner to support you.

Excellent Plant-Based Resources Online

- Nutrition Facts (https://nutritionfacts.org)
- The Physicians Committee for Responsible Medicine (https://www.pcrm.org)
- Forks Over Knives (https://www.forksoverknives.com)
- Happy Cow (https://www.happycow.net)
- VegNews (https://vegnews.com)
- The Plantrician Project (https://plantricianproject.org)
- American College of Lifestyle Medicine (https://www.lifestylemedicine.org)
- eCornell Plant-Based Certificate Program (https://www.ecornell.com/certificates/nutrition/plant-based-nutrition/)

DON'T FEEL LIKE YOU HAVE TO GO COLD TOFURKY (UNLESS YOU REALLY WANT TO)

No question, a whole-food, plant-based diet is the best way to go. But you don't have to do it this very minute. In fact, I never encourage people to go cold turkey (or *tofurky* as plant-based folks like to say) unless they really want to, of course. For a select few with strong wills and good reading habits, it can work. Changing your diet is a learning process, the goal being not just to eat better but to become smarter about your life's choices. You're not just changing your diet; you're changing your whole life. That is scary for a lot of people. Going cold tofurky does not necessarily give you the foundation you need to understand *why* you are doing what you are doing.

So start off with, say, meatless Mondays. Then maybe add to those Mondays no more processed foods as well. Think of this as nutritional basic training. Maybe start learning how to create a tasty, healthy meal that you can then cook again and again. Start learning about new vegetables, fruits, spices, and herbs. Master them. Begin adding meatless Tuesdays and then Wednesdays. Before long, it could be meatless weekdays. You can try going meatless at home while you still eat some animal-based products at restaurants. Eventually you'll find your taste buds will change, you will feel—and be—healthier, and you will actually *want* to go plant based seven days week.

In other words, if you go plant based in small bites, you will have time to digest the process. You will understand why you are eating this way, and that knowledge will help you stay on the right path. Someone telling you not to eat something is not as powerful as you fully understanding why you shouldn't be eating that product.

Moreover, when most people try something new, they start off with great energy—and then fall off the wagon. That's why most diets fail: people get all excited, lose a few pounds, and then lose interest. But if you combine your new diet with knowledge, you'll stay on the path long enough to see results—and results do happen quickly when you follow this plan. As you read already, within three weeks my vision returned, and I was diabetes-free within months. You may not have such a dramatic triumph, but once you get on the bandwagon, you will soon be singing a new tune.

Seven Substitutes for Meat

- **Jackfruit**: A kind of tree related to fig and bread-fruit trees, jackfruit is native to Asia. Its fruit tastes tropical, not unlike pineapple or mango, but when cooked, it tastes almost exactly like pulled pork. And, unlike meat, it is a good source of vitamin C, potassium, and fiber, and is loaded with antioxidants and phytonutrients (chemicals found in plants that help enhance immunity, among other health benefits).

- **Lentils**: These are not only high in protein and fiber while low in fat but resemble ground beef and mix well with many sauces and flavors. One lentil burger and you may be hooked for life. Best of all, they're so cheap you can eat them every day and save your health and money.

- **Mushrooms**: Besides being low in calories and sodium and cholesterol-free, mushrooms are filled with vitamins, minerals, and fiber. They make for a terrific meat substitute, as they are rich, earthy, and feature the taste known as *umami*. You can cook up everything from mushroom Bolognese to portobello mushroom burgers to mushroom bacon bits.

- **Nuts**: Like mushrooms, nuts are an excellent replacement for actual meat. Besides being rich in vitamins and minerals, they can help reduce the risk of many chronic diseases, including diabetes, heart disease, and colon cancer. One recent study from the Harvard School of Public Health showed that replacing one serving of red meat with one serving of nuts reduces mortality risk by 19 percent. Serve up some walnut tacos or vegan nut loaf and be amazed at their meatiness.[1]

- **Seitan** (pronounced say-tan): This tasty morsel is made from wheat, which is why it's known as "wheat meat." By itself it can taste rather bland, like chicken, but when prepared with sauces, it can taste like almost anything you want it to. Seitan is high in protein and an excellent source of minerals like selenium and iron. You can make anything from seitan kebabs with peanut sauce to Philly seitan steak sandwiches. Wherever there was meat, there is seitan.

- **Tempeh:** Made from soybeans that have been fermented and mixed into a dense loaf, tempeh is high in protein, low in fat, and filled with vitamins and minerals. It's becoming more and more popular, as it has a nutty taste that mixes well with many other flavors. Think tempeh teriyaki, tempeh bacon, tempeh veggie stir-fry . . . the possibilities are endless.

- **Tofu:** Another soybean-based food, tofu is made by solidifying soy milk and pressing it into blocks. It comes in many varieties, from extra firm to soft, so it can be used in countless appetizers, entrees, and desserts. Like tempeh, tofu is loaded with protein and is an excellent source of many minerals, such as iron, calcium, phosphorous, and selenium.

SMILE AND LAUGH

Here's something you can try tomorrow: Start and end your day with a smile and a laugh.

Does this seem overly simple? Maybe it is, but laughter isn't just fun; there's a reason the cliché "laughter is the best medicine" has persisted for so many years.

When we laugh, we embrace the true joys of life. I used to wake up in the morning and fret about all the things on my agenda. I'd push myself out of bed with a frown and tell myself that all I wanted to do was just get through the day. Now when I wake up, I immediately put on a smile and start thinking about all the joys the day might bring, all the exciting things I might do, all the new things I might learn.

Doing this every morning has truly changed my day. My days are hectic—sometimes I have to attend a dozen or more meetings and supervise multiple projects. But while I used to see all these tasks as burdens, now I see them as opportunities to meet a goal, learn something new, experience a new thought, meet a new contact. I find a way to smile. I find a way to laugh. And I get others to laugh as well.

Life isn't as serious as we think. When I review some of the most traumatic moments of my life, I can't even see why I was so stressed. If you see yourself through the lens of laughter, you can deal with your past and your present with greater ease and function.

The truth is, laughter is a more serious matter than most people believe. According to the Mayo Clinic, laughter has real and beneficial effects on the body. It can enhance your intake of oxygen and stimulate your heart, lungs, and muscles. It can soothe tension, reduce the physical symptoms of stress, and improve circulation. It can also improve your immune system by releasing stress-fighting neuropeptides. Laughter can lighten physical pain by releasing endorphins in the brain. It can even relieve mental pain by improving your mood faster than a pill, which is something we can all always profit from.

So laugh whenever you can (and when it's appropriate, of course). The lighter your mental burden, the lighter your day. The lighter your day, the more you enjoy everything you do, and that includes your new, healthy diet.

MAKING THE SWITCH

EAT A PLANT-BASED DIET

Of all the steps you can take to good health, this is, by far, the most important. This is where you start. This is where you end. You eat a plant-based diet.

What is a plant-based diet? It's very simple. It's simply one in which you do not eat any animal products. Nothing that ever had a face or a mother. No eggs, no meat, no fish, no shrimp, no cheese. Instead, you eat the best food that Mother Nature has to offer: fruits, vegetables, legumes, and whole grains, which you can eat either cooked or, as some people do, raw.

With these ingredients you can create delicious, mouth-watering meals that will give you all the protein, fat, and carbohydrates your body needs every day.

Before I ate plant based, like most people my meals centered around meats and dairy and processed foods. A meal wasn't complete without meat, not to mention heaps of salt and processed sugar. Breakfast was always eggs; processed meat like sausage, bacon, or ham; some form of sweet Danish pastry; and a glass of orange or cranberry juice. Lunch was more of the same: meat, some kind of pastry on the go, and a sugary beverage. I had a salad now and then, but it was always drenched in fatty, sugary dressing. Dinner was no different: meat, fish, or chicken, usually from a fast-food establishment and often fried; white processed bread; French fries; and a truckload of sugar and salt. I couldn't leave out dessert, of course: ice cream and more pastries, pie, cake, or donuts. No, it's not a myth: cops like donuts.

Today my plant-based diet is just as filling, but far more satisfying. It contains fewer calories and much more health. I start my day with different types of fruits, including a quarter of an apple, an orange, a pear, a slice of mango, a quarter of a grapefruit, and a few cherries. I make a smoothie with a half-cup of blackberries and blueberries, along with broccoli, spinach, and kale. Then I add some ginger and half a teaspoon of carob powder, along with a teaspoon each of acai, amla, moringa, and maca powders. This not only fills me up for hours, it takes away that emotional lull that I always felt after eating all that fried and processed food. I used to feel excited before eating breakfast, but afterward I felt guilty and queasy. These days I still feel excited before eating, but nourished and happy afterward.

For lunch my go-to meal is a blended soup made with a base of black lentils mixed with onion and healthy spices, such as cinnamon, turmeric, and ginger. Then I take a handful of kale, red onions, beets, red cabbage, mushrooms, and carrots and mix them together into the soup. Depending on my mood, sometimes I want the soup to be thick; other times I prefer it thin. Or I make an acai bowl with bananas, peanuts, walnuts, berries, and fruits. That can also be my dinner.

Other times I make a bread out of flaxseed and sweet potatoes and eat it with hummus, or perhaps I just mix up a spinach salad with added hummus.

No more soda, ever! My beverage of choice is water, although sometimes I'll go for seltzer. I do drink cold-brewed tea now and then. (I even eat the leaves with my tea! Why not? They're tasty and good for you. For more, see the Drink Well section on page 76.)

Dessert means chopped up frozen bananas mixed with other frozen fruits and a little almond milk to give it a nice creamy texture. Sometimes I add an avocado to create an amazing rich texture, and maybe some crushed walnuts for taste.

I've ditched the donuts. Now, at snack time, I enjoy walnuts, fruit, and perhaps a date. (Dates are so sugary that I often just cut one in half and eat the other half later.) Alternatively I'll opt for a fig. Both dates and figs satisfy a sugar craving, and both are rich in vitamins and micronutrients.

Before I became plant based, I never would have believed that eating this way would satisfy me. If it wasn't on the dollar menu, or if it wasn't something my mom cooked, then I didn't want anything to do with it. Oh, how wrong I was. Today, eating plant-based food leaves me full and happy due to the fiber content. I feel ready to take on the world, whereas my old diet just made me want to take a nap.

I am also surprised by how much my taste buds have changed. I used to think that a good meal meant lots of sugar, salt, and fat. I had no idea what vegetables and fruits truly tasted like because what few I ate were drowned in sauces and oil. This is one of the most surprising benefits of a plant-based diet: you get your taste buds back!

Note that each person's taste buds are unique. As you discover new foods and new tastes, you'll also discover new ways to make your meals exciting. One of my favorite discoveries was that I love putting small pieces of chopped pears in my soups. This makes me happy, but it might not work for you. As you progress, you'll constantly be taking your foods to the next level and discovering what your taste buds love and don't love. I am still on that journey and always will be. For example, I recently discovered a vegan egg-substitute product called JUST Egg, and now I love to make a sandwich using it and flaxseed bread. I also love some of the new bite-size snacks made from kale and walnuts.

Never stop finding new ways to add healthy foods into your repertoire! And remember: if you're going to succeed at your new plant-based diet, your food must look good, taste good, and be good for you.

AVOID PROCESSED FOODS

One of the cardinal rules of eating healthy: stop stuffing your belly with empty calories and start filling it with nutrients.

Among the first things I learned during my plant-based journey is that just because a food is technically *vegan* doesn't necessarily make it *healthy*. A plant-based diet could consist of potato chips, diet soda, pretzels, popcorn, root beer, and French fries. Totally plant based—and totally unhealthy.

Eating healthy means eating healthy foods. For the most part, this means choosing foods that are as close to their original form as possible. This means potatoes instead of French fries. Tomatoes instead of ketchup. Unsweetened hibiscus tea instead of Kool-Aid. (Hibiscus tea is the OG West African red drink!) Foods lose their nutritional value and get increasingly unhealthy whenever you process them—that is, when you take ingredients out or add ingredients in.

Going Raw

Some folks might go as far as to say that cooking is a form of processing and prefer to eat their veggies raw. That style of eating is called a raw food diet. As for me, I firmly believe that many foods are much better cooked, both taste- and health-wise. Cooked foods are more easily digested, the heat can kill harmful bacteria, and cooking can increase the antioxidant capacity of certain foods, especially tomatoes and carrots.

What's wrong with processed foods? They tend to be filled with chemicals, additives, and other nonnatural ingredients. For instance, many packaged foods have extra sugar in the form of high-fructose corn syrup and other sweet, nonnutritious empty calories. These foods often make you want to eat more than you should by messing with your brain.

Foods filled with these additives are also low in fiber content, which is as important to your diet as vitamins and nutrients. Fiber lowers your cholesterol levels along with your risk of type 2 diabetes, heart disease, and many cancers. (It also reduces the risk of hemorrhoids! For more information about eating enough fiber, see page 74.)

Processed foods make you gain weight—a lot of weight. In an experiment conducted at the National Institutes of Health, researchers discovered that people ate about 500 extra calories per day when their diet was composed mostly of processed foods, compared with people who were given minimally processed foods.

Finally, processed foods are incredibly addictive. Do you remember that famous Lay's Potato Chips ad that gloated, "Betcha can't eat just one?" The ad was correct. Most people can't stop eating added salt, sugars, and fats. Don't be an addict. Kick the habit. Whenever you can, eat foods that are as unprocessed as possible.

UNEARTH NEW FRUITS AND VEGETABLES

Don't laugh: one of my biggest surprises on my journey to health was learning that ketchup is not a vegetable.

I honestly believed that I was partially fulfilling my daily requirement of vegetables based on my consumption of ketchup (which, by the way, is overloaded with sugar and salt). The rest of my vegetable intake was quite small: usually just collard greens and iceberg lettuce (which is basically just water). The collards themselves were quite healthy—that is, until I slathered them in oil and salt. If I did occasionally eat other vegetables, I doused them in as much fat and salt as possible to make them taste like, well, fat and salt.

When I went plant based, I took it upon myself to learn about the dozens of vegetables I had heard about but had never eaten. For one, I kept reading about kale. What the heck was that? A college somewhere in New England? I decided to try it. I didn't like it. Then I learned that if you cooked it right, which I hadn't done, kale could actually be delicious. It turns out that kale is genuine soul food, prepared in dozens of delicious ways by West African cooks.

I next discovered broccoli, bok choy, Brussels sprouts, and other vegetables that I never bothered to eat before. The dam broke. I was soon eating mushrooms, carrots, asparagus, sweet potatoes, red cabbage, beans, peas, and more. I also found that healthy foods I used to dislike, such as onions, could taste excellent if prepared properly. Potatoes, too, could be a good source of nutrients, but only if you prepare them correctly—that is, without deep-frying them into French fries or baking them with sour cream and bacon.

I also used my new knowledge of spices to make these foods work rather than depending on loads of oil and salt. And I learned how to sauté foods in a healthy way, using a combination of lemon and vinegar that gave me the nice salty taste I love without turning them into a diabetes-inducing, artery-clogging nightmare.

Here's a tip: instead of preparing the vegetables each time you eat, cut them up and put them in zip-top bags or food storage containers so that when you're ready to add them to a dish, they're ready to go.

Here are 10 excellent vegetables you might not be eating that add taste and nutrition to your diet:

1. **Beet greens**: Even if you don't like beets, eat the leaves. They're loaded with vitamins and nutrients, including iron, protein, calcium, magnesium, zinc, and fiber. They're low in fat, calories, and cholesterol, and are a great source of fiber. And, of course, they taste great.

2. **Bell peppers**: Well, these are technically fruits because they have seeds, but most people treat them like vegetables. How many foods come in as full a range of colors as peppers? Red, orange, yellow, green—they're all good for you, low in calories, and a great source of vitamins A and C as well as potassium, folate, iron, and fiber. Little known fact: a cup of chopped red bell peppers contains nearly three times more vitamin C than an orange. You can eat peppers raw like you'd eat a fruit or cook them up to complement any number of other foods.

3. **Bok choy**: This Chinese cabbage is another one of those vegetables I'd never heard of, but it's packed with fiber; vitamins C, K, B_6, and A; and beta carotene. It's also a great source of folate and calcium. You can cook it as a side dish or throw its leaves into salads and sandwiches.

4. **Broccoli rabe**: A member of the turnip family, this is loaded with fiber and vitamins—A, C, and K, to name a few—and minerals like calcium, folate, and iron. It's best when cooked, but you can also use it in a salad for a delicious earthy taste.

5. **Fermented vegetables**: These foods, filled with good bacteria, help your gut stay healthy, improve your digestion, boost your immunity, and help you maintain your weight. Many are rich in probiotics. I love all kinds of fermented vegetables, from carrots to green beans. They'll give your taste buds a zippy treat and your stomach a helpful boost.

6. **Kale:** This has gone from a forgotten vegetable to one of the most common in a very short time. The reason kale has become so popular is that it cooks well with many other foods, tastes great in a salad, and is excellent for you. Like these other veggies, it contains a wealth of health, including fiber, antioxidants, calcium, iron, and vitamins K and C.

7. **Microgreens:** They may sound small, but these plants pack a punch. Harvested before they have a chance to grow into their larger form, microgreens contain copious amounts of nutrients, including potassium, iron, zinc, magnesium, copper, and cancer-fighting antioxidants. Some of the healthiest are broccoli, kale, peas, radishes, and arugula.

8. **Seaweed:** Not something most of us ever thought of eating, seaweed is an excellent food—low in fat, high in fiber, and a terrific source of vitamins A, C, E, K, and B, along with minerals, such as iodine, selenium, and iron. You can eat seaweed as flakes poured onto your salads or cereals, stir it into dressings, or you can even toss it into your smoothies.

9. **Sweet potatoes:** These are another excellent source of fiber and are filled with minerals, including iron, selenium, and calcium, and a large array of B and C vitamins. And sweet potatoes are very high in the antioxidant beta-carotene. Many people only eat them at Thanksgiving, but they're far too delicious to enjoy only once a year. Eat them often. They won't bust your budget, either.

10. **Swiss chard:** Another West African soul-food staple, Swiss chard is brimming with vitamins like K, A, and C, and minerals, such as magnesium, potassium, iron, and fiber. You can sauté it, bake it, cream it, or put it in salads and soups. Once you fall in love with Swiss chard, you'll be looking for any excuse to cook with it.

◻ ◻ ◻

Just like with vegetables, I never gave fruit much of a chance. At best I was an apple-a-day guy. But it didn't keep the doctor away. Now every morning, along with my smoothie, I have a quarter of an apple, an orange, a peach, a nectarine, a quarter of a banana, a few cherries, strawberries, blueberries, and any in-season berries.

Learning about all kinds of wonderful nutritious fruits has been one of the best parts of my journey to good health. Here are some other fruits you might want to try:

- **Cherimoya:** Native to South America, this is also called a custard apple because that's what it tastes like. It's a great source of vitamins B and C and is chock-full of fiber. If you don't believe me, take it from Mark Twain, who called the cherimoya "the most delicious fruit known to man."

- **Durian:** Okay, bad news first: durian smells awful. Like really awful. The good news? It tastes *nothing* like its odor. Native to tropical regions, durian is known in Southeast Asia as the "king of fruits." If you don't mind the odor, you'll get a fruit that combines the taste of vanilla with bananas. It's rich in fiber and minerals like manganese, iron, and copper, and is a great source of B vitamins as well.

- **Fuyu persimmon:** Crisp and sweet, few fruits are as tasty as this kind of persimmon, which, unlike its relatives, is not astringent. You can eat the skin if you'd like, although many people don't. It's an excellent source of fiber as well as vitamins A, C, and B_6, along with minerals like potassium and manganese.

- **Kumquat:** A superb source of vitamin C and fiber, this citrus fruit is also rich in the powerful antioxidant beta carotene. And it's got lots of calcium to keep your bones strong. Because it can taste slightly sour (unlike its skin, which is sweet), it makes an excellent marmalade.

- **Passion fruit:** Native to South America, this fruit is, like so many others, loaded with fiber and vitamins C and A and is rich in antioxidants. It tastes like a mix of many other tropical fruits, such as pineapple, papaya, mango, citrus, and guava.

- **Pawpaw:** Most of the other fruits here come from exotic places of the world, but the pawpaw is native to North America. Oddly it tastes more like a tropical fruit than other American ones, something between a banana and a pineapple. Pawpaws are high in vitamin C as well as minerals like magnesium, iron, copper, manganese, and zinc.

- **Pomelo:** Native to South America, this citrus fruit could be mistaken for a sweet version of a grapefruit. Surprisingly high in protein—one fruit contains 4.6 grams—it is also a superb source of vitamin C while offering healthy amounts of thiamin, riboflavin, niacin, and vitamin B_6.

EAT WHOLE

Our bodies are not one-size-fits-all. For example, eating a banana spikes my sugar levels, while another person can eat three bananas and barely see an effect. All we know is that certain foods are universally bad for everyone, although they harm us in different ways. Plant foods, on the other hand, are universally good for us—with a few exceptions.

For instance, among some people, grains can cause unusual reactions, from bloating to allergies to more serious complications. Everyone who tries a plant-based diet needs to test their reaction to whole grains. Although there are many diets out there touting the advantages of cutting grains out altogether, such as the nutritionally disastrous keto diet or the nearly as bad paleo diet, the most sound research has shown that whole grains are indeed a necessary part of a healthy diet.

What are whole grains? They are seeds of grasses known collectively as cereals, the most popular being wheat, rice, and corn. Less well-known, yet just as nutritious, are quinoa and amaranth. There are many grains to pick from, but only pick those that are whole, meaning their germ (the inner layer) and their bran (the outer layer) have not been removed. For example, this means picking brown rice over white rice. When you remove the germ and bran, you're left with the endosperm—the part that is most filled with empty carbohydrates and not the essential vitamins, fiber, protein, and minerals. When you eat these whole grains, you lower your risk of heart disease, stroke, obesity, type 2 diabetes, certain cancers, and countless other chronic conditions.

Of course, the other issue to keep in mind: avoid processed grains. Even though they are technically vegan, processed grains aren't healthy foods. This means you have to be very careful when you shop. Food producers like to trick you by adding brown food coloring to their bread and calling it multigrain. Don't fall for these meaningless slogans. You want whole and nothing but whole. I know many people who have a big smile on their face when they tell me they eat their multigrain toast every morning. I hate to tell them that they are not doing themselves any favors; multi does not mean whole. It just means a lot of different processed grains.

I eat whole grains often, but seldom in large quantities because I like to diversify my diet. But if I eat bread, it will be whole grain. If I eat oatmeal, it will be steel cut (which is less processed than rolled oats). Whatever grains I eat, they're 100 percent whole, no exceptions.

Gluten

A small number of people suffer from celiac disease, which is an allergic reaction to gluten-containing foods, such as wheat, barley, and rye. If you are one of these people, you should skip the gluten grains and instead choose ones that are gluten-free, such as quinoa and oats.

Generally speaking, if you don't have celiac disease, there is no reason to avoid gluten. Unfortunately some associate *gluten* with *unhealthy*, which is simply not the case. A very small amount of people who do not have celiac disease also seem to have a negative reaction to gluten, but it is not clear why. In fact, a study in the journal *Digestion* found that 86 percent of people who thought they were gluten sensitive actually were not. In truth, only 1 percent of Americans suffer from celiac disease.

SKIP THE OIL

Even though they are technically plant based, cooking oils are un-healthy. They are also wasteful: it takes about 40 olives just to make one tablespoon of olive oil, for example. On top of that, you're not getting any of the fiber those 40 olives would provide had you con-sumed them whole.

Olive oil is also pure fat, to the tune of 14 grams per table-spoon. Some people claim that this is "good fat," but I don't buy it. It's just too much fat to be good! Many of the doctors I admire, such as Dr. Caldwell Esselstyn, Jr., strongly recommend weaning yourself off oil, especially if you suffer from heart disease or dia-betes. Oil is harmful to the endothelium, which is the innermost lining of the artery. Injury to the endothelium, he says, is the gateway to vascular disease.

Your body needs essential fatty acids, but you don't need oil to get them. They can be found in everything from green leafy vege-tables, flaxseeds, and soybeans to nuts and seeds. A wide-ranging whole-food, plant-based diet provides the fatty acids you need, without the worry of the possible health issues associated with processed oils.

But how do you cook without oil? There are plenty of ways to cook without using it. I love to sauté my vegetables, but instead of oil I use water, broth, or wine. If I'm baking bread, I use apple sauce, a squashed banana, or a sweet potato. There are countless products that give me the same results that oil provides. I am also a fan of the hot-air fryer, which I use when I want that deep-fried taste without the unhealthy deep fry.

Not-Very-Virgin Oil

Think that your oil is healthy because it's labeled "extra-virgin"? In theory, extra-virgin olive oil is the healthiest because it undergoes the least processing. There are no solvents and other chemicals added that degrade the oil under high temperatures. However, while the more expensive extra-virgin olive oil is certainly the best kind of olive oil, that doesn't make it healthy. You are still consuming liquid fat; it's just not laced with chemicals.

And, in reality, much of what we think is "extra-virgin" olive oil really isn't. Studies show that up to 70 percent of so-called extra-virgin olive oil is actually diluted with much cheaper oils.

EAT YOUR FIBER

One of the most important areas of health is your digestive system, and although people are more than happy to talk about stomach aches, they don't feel comfortable talking about issues like constipation or anything else involving the toilet. But how can you discuss health in your body without talking about what comes out of your body?

There's nothing in us that should be shameful or taboo to talk about. Yet we don't talk about issues like women's menstrual cycles, impotence, or our bathroom habits. In order to stay healthy, we must have these discussions. We have to embrace their importance. We have to teach our children—and everyone else—to feel comfortable bringing up these topics. In other words, your poop says a great deal about your health.

Unfortunately people have normalized the idea of constipation. I have some friends who think it's perfectly fine to have bowel movements every few days. They just assume everyone feels as stuffed and bloated as they do.

Not so.

One of the most wonderful parts of a plant-based diet is that you will learn that you can have daily, easy bowel movements. You may not talk about them much to others, but you will certainly say to yourself how happy you are not to feel constipated anymore.

How do you become so regular? By eating plant food filled with fiber. Fiber is the part of your diet that makes your digestive system act like a superhighway: everything flows the way it should.

What is fiber? Also sometimes called bulk, it is the indigestible parts of the plants you are now eating and loving. Without fiber in your diet, you put yourself at more risk for all kinds of conditions, from cancer to cardiac issues, from diabetes to obesity.

There are two kinds of fiber: soluble and insoluble. Soluble means that it dissolves in water. Insoluble means it does not. Both are necessary. Soluble fiber helps lower your cholesterol and your blood sugar levels and improves your immune system. Insoluble fiber is terrific for making your bowel movements a pleasure and helps prevent colon cancer and other digestive diseases.

Plant-based foods are the only source of fiber in nature. That's right, you can't get any from meat, dairy, eggs, or fish. Unfortunately 97 percent of Americans are fiber deficient, which means that 97 percent of Americans aren't eating enough plants. No, white bread does not count. You need to eat whole fruits, vegetables, grains, and—most important—beans to take in the amount of fiber necessary to stay regular and to stay healthy.

Great Sources of Fiber

- **Soluble fiber**: oatmeal, beans, lentils, apples, blueberries, Brussels sprouts, spinach, oranges, prunes
- **Insoluble fiber**: whole wheat, cauliflower, tomatoes, carrots, dark green leafy vegetables, nuts, seeds

Because I eat so much fiber-rich food, I don't need to sit down and count how much of it I am consuming. I eat so many fruits, vegetables, beans, legumes, and whole grains that I know I'm getting enough!

How much fiber should you eat? It varies by age and gender: Men 50 and younger should consume 38 grams a day; men who are older can get by with 30. Women 50 and younger need 25 grams daily, while those older than 50 need 21 grams.

It's best not to get bogged down with numbers, though. If you're eating a whole-food, plant-based diet every day, you are getting enough fiber. It's as easy as that.

MAKE YOUR GUT HAPPY

Your gut is an amazing place. It's basically your body's second brain, a place with a nervous system all its own, containing more than 100 million nerve cells. It's one you've definitely felt from time to time, like when you're nervous and get butterflies in your stomach. Science is still trying to figure out everything the gut can do, but we do know that it plays a critical role in our health, particularly due to all the bacteria residing within it.

First off, what is the gut? It encompasses your entire digestive system, but usually, when we say gut, we're really talking about your large intestine (which is quite large at five feet long). Within it are not only those 100 million nerve cells, but also trillions—yes, trillions with a T—of microorganisms.

These bacteria not only affect how your food is digested, they also affect your heart rhythms; they help produce certain vitamins, such as B vitamins and K; they help lower your risk of diabetes and cancer; and they can lower (or raise) your weight. Too few bacteria in your gut may also wreak havoc on your immune system. And this is just scratching the surface of what we know so far. Our guts have many more secrets to teach us.

Now, not all bacteria are good. When your gut bacteria are out of balance, you can come down with serious digestive conditions, such as irritable bowel syndrome and leaky gut syndrome.

How do you make sure that your gut is healthy and filled with trillions of happy inhabitants? You guessed it: eat a plant-based diet. When your diet is high in animal protein, salt, alcohol, and artificial sweeteners, your gut suffers. When you eat a plant-based diet, your bacteria flourishes. It's as simple as that.

What are the best foods to ensure a healthy gut? Fermented foods top the list: kimchi (a Korean dish made of fermented cabbage), yogurt (with a nondairy base, such as soy, coconut, or cashew), lentils, nuts, bananas, onions, garlic (which has so many healthy qualities), and apples.

By the way, there are numerous non-diet related ways to harm your gut bacteria, such as a lack of physical exercise, smoking cigarettes, stress, and sleeplessness. Remember, good health is more than just a terrific diet. It's a terrific lifestyle.

DRINK WELL

When you're living a healthy lifestyle, you're not just thinking about what you eat. What you drink matters too. Before I started my health journey, I drank lots and lots of ginger ale. I loved it. Sugary, spicy ginger ale. I also was fond of orange juice, which may sound healthy, but is mainly just sugar. I did drink water too, but that wasn't my go-to drink.

Now when I'm thirsty, I choose seltzer or plain water, or I reach for some healthy red drink: cold-brewed hibiscus tea. It not only tastes terrific, but it's loaded with antioxidants, may lower your blood pressure, and is good for your liver.

It's crucial to hydrate throughout your day with beverages as healthy as your food. The old saying goes you need to drink eight glasses of water a day, which is generally a good rule of thumb. (Technically the National Academies of Sciences, Engineering, and Medicine recommend about 15 cups for men and 11 cups for women.) Not any liquid will do, though. An old police friend used to brag that he always drank eight mugs of cola every day. Not good.

So don't think eight glasses of liquids. Think *water*. Another friend on the force boasted about how much juice she drank. Also not good. Fruit juices are loaded with sugar, and unlike eating fruit, you are not getting any fiber. Remember fiber? It's your friend! The juicing process removes all the healthy fiber and leaves you with sugar water. (As an alternative to juicing, try smoothies, which keep the fiber intact.)

When you eat a plant-based diet, you are consuming many foods with a high water content, so don't worry too much about hitting eight glasses per day. And remember, we're all different, with varying weights, activity levels, and metabolism. Only your body can truly say how much water you need. As always, be sensible, be practical, be smart, and when in doubt, find an authoritative source and read up. Never stop learning!

What about Alcohol?

Everyone knows that water is good for us. But what about alcohol? It seems every other day there is a new study saying that a glass of wine per day is good for us. Or that it's terrible for us.

The truth is we don't know for sure, but the science is clear that too much alcohol is very bad for us, raising the risk of everything from heart disease to obesity to breast, colon, and pancreatic cancers. To be on the safe side, I try to avoid alcohol except for special occasions, when I like to sip some single-malt whiskey.

So if you're hankering for a beer, maybe try making a smoothie instead.

CUT THE SALT AND SUGAR

We've talked a lot about animal fat and protein in this book but not much about salt.

Most people know that consuming too much salt, also called sodium, can lead to high blood pressure. That's because too much sodium in your blood hinders your kidneys from removing excess water, increasing your blood pressure and straining your delicate blood vessels, leading to heart disease.

Nevertheless, most Americans still consume far too much of it. Sure, salt makes everything taste better, but enough already! The truth is, food often tastes better without salt; it was only when I stopped relying on salt that I began to truly taste the wonderful flavors of my favorite vegetables and legumes. Until then, I thought most vegetables tasted the same because, well, they all tasted kind of salty. Studies show that salt blunts our taste buds over time, so it might take some time to acclimate yourself to the way food is *supposed* to taste. Fear not! Just like you can slowly wean yourself off animal food, you can slowly wean yourself off salt.

It's important to note that while too much of it is bad, salt is still a necessary nutrient. We need sodium (which makes up about

40 percent of salt; the other 60 percent is chloride) in our diet. The good news is that plant foods have plenty of naturally occurring sodium, so you can eventually toss away that saltshaker for good.

As for recreating that salty taste, I've found that a combination of vinegar with lemon is a fantastic way to accent my food without busting my arteries.

Foods That Contain Surprising Amounts of Sodium

- Breakfast cereals (one cup of Kellogg's Raisin Bran has 210 milligrams)
- Canned vegetables (one 4.5 ounce jar of Green Giant Sliced Mushrooms has 570 milligrams)
- Canned soups (one can of Campbell's Chunky Savory Vegetable Soup has—yes—1,680 milligrams)
- Ketchup (154 milligrams per tablespoon)
- Salad dressings (depending on the variety, about 134 milligrams per tablespoon)
- Bread (one pita may have as much as 500 milligrams)
- Soy sauce (879 milligrams per tablespoon)
- Processed cheeses (one slice of Kraft Singles has 220 milligrams)
- Cottage cheese (up to 400 milligrams per half cup)
- Instant oatmeal (more than 200 milligrams in a packet)
- Veggie burgers (one Beyond Burger patty has 350 milligrams)

Just like with salt, Americans are *bombarded* with sugar. Everywhere we go, everything we do, everything we eat: there's sugar, sugar, sugar. I remember talking to a French friend of mine who is a pastry chef; he said that it was extremely difficult to create his desserts in America because he had to double the sweetness in comparison with other countries.

The American palette demands sugar. But sugar is like a drug, so the more we eat, the more our tongue gets desensitized to the taste, which means we want more and more—until we come down with a serious condition. Sugar can hurt us in many ways, from weight gain to acne to increased risk of heart disease, diabetes, and cancer. That's just the start. Sugar can even contribute to symptoms of depression, harm our livers, cause tooth decay, and deplete our energy. And it's not easy to give up, either. Studies show that eating sugar can cause the brain to release dopamine, a neurotransmitter associated with the pleasure and reward centers of the brain—just like with narcotics. Some scientists even consider sugar to be more addictive than cocaine.

And don't be fooled by other names for sugar, such as high-fructose corn syrup, raw sugar, liquid sugar, and brown sugar. And be particularly careful if you do choose to eat canned or processed foods as they can be even higher in sugar than soda. Food manufacturers even bake sugar into bread to make it more addictive.

Sneaky Names for Sugar

- Barley malt
- Cane juice
- Corn syrup
- Dextran and dextrose
- Fructose
- Rice syrup
- Honey
- Lactose
- Malt
- Maple syrup
- Molasses

The lesson here: just like with animal protein, just like with salt, it's time to wean yourself off sugar. There are other, much more healthy ways to satisfy a sweet tooth. As for me, I love dates. They not only taste terrific, they are high in fiber, loaded with antioxidants, and filled with nutrients, such as potassium, magnesium, and iron, among many others. Another great choice for a sugar rush is figs. Like dates, figs are bursting with fiber along with potassium, calcium, and iron and antioxidants like vitamins A and K.

One of my favorite ways to placate the occasional need for something sweet is to chop up a small piece of fruit and add it to soup; you'd be amazed how well that sweet little morsel completely changes what you thought was boring old soup.

And every now and then I indulge in a dessert, but I'm not talking about brownies and cakes. For starters, try a delicious homemade vegan ice cream: simply freeze bananas and then put them into a blender; add walnuts and frozen berries and blend. You can add some oat or almond milk for texture if you'd like. For other dessert possibilities, see page 175.

Foods That Contain Surprising Amounts of Sugar

- Low-fat yogurt (a single cup can contain up to 47 grams of sugar)
- Pasta sauce (between 6 to 12 grams of sugar per half cup)
- Granola bars (between 8 to 12 grams per bar)
- Barbecue sauce (2 tablespoons can contain up to 15 grams of sugar)
- Ketchup (just 1 tablespoon contains 1 teaspoon of sugar)
- Iced tea (most commercially prepared iced teas contain around 33 grams of sugar per 12-ounce serving, similar to a can of cola)
- Dried fruit (a small box of raisins contains about 25 grams of sugar)
- Coleslaw (10 grams of sugar reside in a normal-size side)
- Canned fruits (most commercially packaged fruits have between 15 and 60 grams of sugar)

FIND WONDERFUL NEW FOODS

When starting a new health plan, people often fear they will be dealing with restrictions. When they hear the word *vegan,* they think: *Even more restrictions.* When I introduce people to a plant-based diet, I try not to begin with all the foods they can't eat. Instead, I emphasize all the new and exciting foods they will start eating.

It's amazing how long I have lived on this planet and yet how little I knew about all the wonderful foods that I could have been eating. I wasn't curious enough to find out what they tasted like because I was so stuck in my routine of meat, potatoes, and fast food. Now my diet is not only diverse but grows more varied and interesting each week.

Take tofu, for instance. I am sure that the mind plays a major role in our taste buds, because if you had told me to try tofu while I was a police officer, I would have said, "I don't eat it, and I don't want to." I thought about the consistency and the taste, and yuck! I couldn't deal with it. But once I opened my mind up to giving new foods a try, wow! Tofu is terrific. It's a major part of my diet because it's healthy, cooks up quickly, and soaks up so many wonderful flavors. I even use it in my desserts, which I never, ever would have thought possible.

Once you fall in love with tofu, you'll fall for tempeh too. Tempeh is fermented tofu, and many nutritionists argue that fermented foods are extremely good for you. Tempeh, like tofu, can be prepared in so many ways that you'll never run out of new dishes to try. My own favorite is tempeh bacon. I put it in sandwiches and in soups, or use it as a meal with a starch, such as rice.

Another excellent substitute for meat that you'll love: seitan. I had never heard of this food, and everyone seems unsure of its pronunciation (say-tan). Seitan is also known as the "wheat meat" because it's made from gluten, which is the primary protein in wheat. Like tofu, seitan makes a wonderful main course, absorbing the flavors and textures of whatever you choose to cook it with. Try a seitan scaloppini and your taste buds will never stop thanking you.

Nutritional yeast is still another food you might not have heard of, but once you've tasted it, you'll wonder where it's been all your life. The name sounds weird, but the taste is great. (Some people shorten the name to "nooch.") Nutritional yeast is what's called a deactivated yeast, and it's sold in the form of yellow powder or flakes. Once upon a time you could find it only in health-food stores, but now it's pretty much everywhere. It has a delicious cheesy taste, so you can use it like grated parmesan. Use it alone or mix it with some ground-up cashews and sprinkle it on snacks, especially popcorn. Or use it on main courses, like pasta.

Still one more food I couldn't for the life of me pronounce: quinoa (keen-wa). Quinoa is a gluten-free plant food that is loaded with antioxidants, fiber, vitamins, minerals, and lots of protein. What's also great is it tastes wonderful and fills you up. You can add it to salads, soups, and cereals; you can make tasty bowls with quinoa and other healthy ingredients; you can mix it into vegan burgers to make them even better. The list of what quinoa can do is as long as your imagination.

So instead of eating the same old unhealthy foods every day, start filling yourself up with all these wonderful new foods that you've probably never tried, or even heard about—foods that will keep hunger (and the doctor) away and give you that wonderfully full feeling you've been craving. What more could you ask for?

PLANNING YOUR MEALS

LEARN ABOUT NUTRITIONAL DENSITY

One of the biggest mistakes you can make with your food is to focus on calories rather than nutrition. How many times have you finished a meal and thought, *Did I eat too many calories? Did I eat too few?*

Stop driving yourself crazy by fretting about calories. Instead, you should be asking yourself: *Is my stomach full of the nutritional foods that my body needs?*

It isn't about being full of food; it's about being full of health.

I like to compare our bodies to a car. You can't just fill the gas tank with any old liquid; you have to fill it with gasoline. Use anything else and you'll be calling a mechanic. That is what happens when you put unhealthy processed food in your body. Your body might chug along for a while, but you'll eventually need to call a mechanic—well, in this case, a doctor—to perform some serious maintenance.

As we've already seen, the good news is the body is capable of healing itself. When you have a steady diet of nutritionally dense meals, you allow your body to dissolve all that plaque, inflammation, and excess fat it has been coping with for years and years. Nutritionally dense foods are those that are high in nutrients but relatively low in calories. They contain a healthy array of vitamins, minerals, complex carbohydrates, and protein.

What are some of the best nutritionally dense foods? You can't beat the cruciferous vegetables: kale, broccoli, cabbage, and cauliflower. Other nutritionally dense foods include spinach, leafy green vegetables, sweet potatoes, garlic, blueberries and strawberries, almonds, tomatoes, asparagus, lentils, and mushrooms.

By the way, it's important not to cook your nutrients away. If you are boiling your foods until they're limp, or frying them to a crisp, they won't supply your body with their best benefits. Learn how to cook with a light touch. Think about a quick stir-fry, or a steam, or even a light spin in the microwave, which retains most of the nutrients.

I always make sure that I have nutritionally dense meals, even when I have little time. For example, my best grab-and-go one is a black bean soup with shredded or chopped kale, spinach, broccoli, red cabbage, red onions, beets, celery, some great seasoning, and cauliflower rice. A big bowl of that and I'm full for hours.

DON'T CONFUSE VEGAN WITH HEALTHY

A vegan friend of mine, Betty, constantly eats out at vegan restaurants. She loves their vegan buffalo wings, vegan steaks, and vegan desserts, but when you actually consider the food she's eating, much of it is processed junk filled with oil, salt, and sugar. Betty's diet is not about nutrients. It's about antinutrients.

Believe it or not, some of the unhealthiest people I know are vegan. Please don't conflate the word *vegan* with *healthy*. Diet soda, graham crackers, Fritos, Twizzlers, soy lattes—all of these may be animal-free, but they've replaced flesh with processed sugar, fat, salt, and a laundry list of chemicals. The result is a diet almost as destructive to your health as an animal-based one.

Just as important as eating vegan food is eating whole foods. Remember, whole foods are ones that have had nothing bad added and nothing good taken away, just as nature intended. The closer you are to whole foods, or foods with limited additives, the healthier you'll be.

SEARCH OUT EXCELLENT, TASTY RECIPES

I tend to think recipes are overrated. I know, I know, there are over 50 delicious recipes at the end of this book that I recommend everyone try. What I mean is that people should not limit themselves to other people's recipes. Use them as a starting point and then experiment. Create your own. Watch as your taste buds adapt and grow and thirst for new foods.

If you don't yet feel confident doing this, go online and search for healthy whole-food, plant-based recipes. You'll find literally thousands. Or go to any bookstore and pick out an excellent vegan cookbook. And, of course, go to Chapter 4 in this book. When you've mastered them, try tweaking the ingredients. Add new vegetables. Substitute tahini sauce for peanut sauce. Take your favorite recipes and combine them into something entirely new.

9 Great Vegan Cookbooks

1. *I Can Cook Vegan* by Isa Chandra Moskowitz
2. *Afro-Vegan* by Bryant Terry
3. *Forks Over Knives—The Cookbook* by Del Sroufe
4. *Vegan Richa's Indian Kitchen* by Richa Hingle
5. *Vegan for Everybody* by America's Test Kitchen
6. *The Homemade Vegan Pantry* by Miyoko Schinner
7. *The Oh She Glows Cookbook* by Angela Liddon
8. *Vegan Planet, Revised Edition* by Robin Robertson
9. *Frugal Vegan* by Katie Koteen and Kate Kasbee

THINK WHOLE FOOD, NOT JUNK FOOD

Here's a good rule of thumb: Avoid foods with more than three ingredients. Once you start going past three, you are eating questionable products that are less a food than a food-like substance.

Whole foods are foods in their most natural state: vegetables, fruits, whole grains, and beans. With a whole food, you can look at it and know what it is.

Consider keeping a daily food log. Every day write down what you had for breakfast, lunch, dinner, and snacks. Then look these items up online. Find out how healthy they are, how whole they are, and how bad they are. Notice how your body reacts to them. Most people don't react well to junk food, but they don't think about it because they've never considered there was a correlation. But you may notice that every time you eat a bag of Cheetos, you get a headache. That every time you down a gallon of soda, your stomach feels bloated. That every time you eat a bucket of fried chicken, you feel lethargic. Your body is telling you it hates these foods; you just aren't listening.

When you get better at adding up the bad versus the good foods you eat, you can also add up all the grams of fat, salt, and sugar (much of which you only find out about when you look at the ingredient list). In addition, you'll be amazed at how much you eat compared to how much you *thought* you ate. For most of us, eating is not something we think about or remember. We just do it. And we don't do it well.

EAT GOOD FAT. DON'T EAT BAD FAT.

Fat is a dirty word these days. Look in the grocery store and you'll see countless products that say "low fat" or "fat free."

Fat isn't necessarily a bad thing. In fact, our bodies need it to survive. (After all, essential fatty acids weren't named *essential* for nothing. They are indeed essential!) Fat helps us absorb many nutrients, such as vitamins A, D, and E (which is why they are known as the fat-soluble vitamins). Fats also produce important hormones, and it is the major form of storage for energy.

There are four kinds of fats, two of which can be healthy and two of which are unhealthy. The healthy ones are monounsaturated and polyunsaturated fats. Studies indicate that these are good to eat in moderation: you can find monounsaturated fat in olives, avocados, peanuts, and almonds. Foods that have polyunsaturated fats include walnuts, sunflower seeds, and flaxseeds. (However, if you are trying to lose weight or reverse your diabetes, you should limit your intake of these fats.)

The first unhealthy fat is saturated fat, which most research shows will raise your cholesterol and cause inflammation. Saturated fats are found mainly in animal products, although a few plant-based foods contain them as well. Coconut oil, for instance, is about 90 percent saturated fat, so don't believe all the supposed heart-healthy hype. Finally, there is trans fat, which is primarily found in foods via an industrial process that converts unsaturated fats to saturated ones. Though they've been mostly banned in this country, trans fats are found naturally in the meat and dairy from cows, sheep, and goats. They form as a by-product when bacteria in the animals' stomachs digest grass.

EDUCATE YOURSELF ABOUT VITAMINS AND MINERALS

FORGET ABOUT PROTEIN

If there's a question I get asked more than any other, it's this: Where do you get your protein? Most people will go on and on about how you have to get protein from meat and eggs. I simply reply, "I get my protein from the same place that cows get theirs: from plants." This is one of the most important messages about eating healthy that we must get across—that everyone can get all the protein they need, and more, from plant-based foods.

We also have to educate people to understand that overconsumption of protein is actually very unhealthy. Our country has a toxically macho perspective on protein. Strong people eat lots of steak, we are conditioned to think. Not true. Strong people are plant strong.

When I was growing up, whenever I would play sports, it was always drummed into me that I had to get plenty of protein to do really well. It was wimpy not to chow down on pounds of meat.

Performance-Enhancing Beets

Athletes are always looking for an edge on the competition. But instead of reaching for those ubiquitous tubs of protein powder, the smart athlete heads to the produce aisle. Specifically, she wants beets.

Beets? Really? you might be thinking. Yes, beets! I know they don't sound like the coolest food in the world, let alone one that makes you run faster, but science backs me up on this one. Check out the name of this study: "Whole Beetroot Consumption Acutely Improves Running Performance." Male and female athletes ate about a cup and a half of baked beets and ran a 5K.[2] Sure enough, during the final mile, the beet group pulled ahead of the control group, who did not dope up with beets beforehand. Not only did the plant-powered athletes run 5 percent faster, their hearts didn't work any harder. So instead of buying the latest $200 pair of Nikes, first try investing in some $2 beets.

When I was growing up, my family's diet centered on our protein source. It wasn't just about the actual food. It was about status. If I went to a friend's house for dinner and his parents didn't put meat on the table, they became the talk of the block. Those people are so poor they can't even afford meat!

Don't think about old-fashioned status symbols; think about the fact that there is protein in literally every fruit, vegetable, and grain.

In actuality, Americans are eating way too much protein—about twice the recommended amount. This is terrible for our health, leading to everything from kidney damage to weight gain, from constipation to an increased cancer risk, from heart disease to calcium loss. The recommended dietary allowance for protein is about 46 grams for women and 54 grams for men. Those levels are incredibly easy to reach on a plant-based diet. It's actually almost impossible to live in America and not get enough protein. In fact, Americans get so much protein in their diet that we don't even have a word for protein deficiency in the English language; we had to borrow it from the Ga language in Ghana. (The word is *kwashiorkor*.)

EAT GREENS FOR CALCIUM

Right after people ask me, "Where do you get your protein," they demand, "Well, where do you get your calcium?"

Before I was heathy, drinking milk was part of my every day. I just knew I had to build a strong body, and a strong body meant strong bones, and that in turn meant that I had to drink almost a quart of milk a day. Milk is the best source of calcium, right? That's what everyone has said for years. When you grow up in the inner city, your food choices are limited, and you get almost no education about nutrition, which means that television ads become the major source of information. We all wanted that famous white mustache to show that we got our milk and calcium.

It's hard to understand what an enormous impact TV has on our health and our food choices. We see countless commercials about how tasty meat is, how healthy milk is, how excellent eggs are—these messages inform and overwhelm us because we see no information from the other side, from the healthy side. When was the last time you saw a commercial that said collard greens are an excellent source of calcium? Big Broccoli doesn't have the same high-powered lobbyists as the National Cattlemen's Beef Association.

When I talk to mothers with young kids, they'll say they've been working to get chocolate milk out of schools because of the sweetness, yet they embrace standard milk; they don't realize how much sugar is in regular milk or how harmful it is for growing boys and girls. Likewise, the seniors I meet with each week tell me that they always drink milk; their doctors told them it's a great way to get calcium and fight osteoporosis.

What we've learned about calcium over the years falls into the category of things that we must *unlearn*. Back when you were growing up, you may have had one or two friends who were lactose intolerant. You probably thought something was wrong with them. But did you know that approximately 65 percent of the human population is lactose intolerant? That means most of us are eating and drinking dairy and putting up with all that bloating, cramping, gas, and diarrhea because we assume it's normal. We're so used to pain that we forget how often we experience it.

Recent studies have also indicated that the proteins in milk may also damage the production of insulin in people who are at a high risk of diabetes and that there may well be a link between milk and prostate cancer. You may be surprised to learn that countries with the highest rates of osteoporosis also have the highest consumption of dairy products.

Instead of drinking milk, try these excellent sources of calcium: bananas, dark green leafy vegetables, broccoli, lentils, tahini, figs, almonds, and tofu. In fact, collard greens are one of the best sources of calcium around. And, it's a healthy source.

PACK VITAMINS AND MINERALS INTO YOUR DIET

Your food should be filled with the best vitamins and minerals possible. The good news is that there's no better way to fill that demand than by eating a plant-based diet.

When I first started my journey to health, I thought I would have to map a program to make sure I got all the appropriate nutrients my body needed. Then, after taking notes, I realized I was getting everything I wanted without even thinking about it. Now I'm on autopilot because my meals are filled with all the nutrition I need.

Vitamin B$_{12}$

A plant-based diet gives you every nutrient you need except one: vitamin B$_{12}$.

As Dr. Neal Barnard explains, "Vitamin B$_{12}$ is not made by plants or animals. It is made by bacteria. Presumably, before the advent of modern hygiene, there were traces of bacteria in the soil and on vegetables and fruits that provided traces of vitamin B$_{12}$. Those days are long gone, of course. Animals have bacteria in their digestive tracts that produce vitamin B$_{12}$, and traces of it end up in meat, dairy products, and eggs. But there are two problems with animal sources. First, they also contain cholesterol, fat, and animal proteins. Second, their absorption is not always sufficient, which is why the US government recommends that everyone over age fifty take a B$_{12}$ supplement."[3]

So, yes, everyone should take a vitamin B$_{12}$ supplement, which is widely available online or at any health-food store. Many people take a weekly 2,000 microgram dose, while Dr. Barnard recommends you take a daily B$_{12}$ supplement using the smallest dose you can find.

Almost all fruits and vegetables are packed with the nutrients you need to live a healthy life. Some may have more than others, although it's hard to go wrong. The following are some of the most nutrient-packed plants around:

- **Spinach**: A great source of iron, vitamins, and antioxidants, spinach is particularly high in vitamin K (an entire daily requirement filled with just one cup) as well as folate and magnesium.

- **Blueberries:** Not only do they taste great, they're little bombs of minerals and vitamins, from C to B_6, from folate to potassium, and the cherry on top of the blueberry is its high fiber content, not to mention its myriad antioxidants.

- **Kale:** In just one cup, kale has only 7 calories, along with copious amounts of vitamins A, C, and K. Kale may even help reduce your cholesterol levels.

- **Black beans:** Technically legumes, not vegetables, black beans are filled with protein (one cup gives you 15 grams) and are an excellent source of fiber and magnesium, which is great for bone health. And they're inexpensive enough to eat every day.

- **Avocados:** Your guacamole not only goes well as a dip for raw veggies, it's a powerhouse of vitamins C, E, K, and B_6 and offers a laundry list of nutrients from folate to niacin. Yes, avocados contain fat, but it's the beneficial monounsaturated variety. While extremely healthy, avocados are high in calories, so eat them in moderation.

- **Broccoli:** Again, all the vitamin K you need in one day, plus twice the daily recommended amount of vitamin C.

- **Peas:** They may look small, but they're mighty. Peas are brimming with vitamins, minerals, antioxidants, phytonutrients, and fiber. Peas may even help reduce your cholesterol levels.

- **Garlic:** It's remarkable how good garlic is for you. Studies indicate eating it can reduce the number of colds you have each year and reduce blood pressure and cholesterol levels. The list of what garlic can do for you is too long to include here, so I encourage you to do some research— Dr. Michael Greger's nutritionfacts.org is a fantastic resource—and you'll be amazed!

- **Cherries:** Another great source of fiber, vitamins, and minerals—especially calcium and potassium—cherries also deliver a considerable helping of antioxidants.

- **Cauliflower:** One of the cruciferous vegetables (along with broccoli, cabbage, bok choy, and Brussels sprouts, among others), cauliflower is high in fiber and B vitamins, low in calories, and filled with antioxidants and phytonutrients. Moreover, a cauliflower steak is one of the heartiest meat substitutes you can cook up.

- **Bell peppers**: A member of the nightshade family (along with tomatoes, also a very healthy choice) and a surprisingly great source of vitamin C (and many other vitamins), peppers are low in calories and rich in antioxidants.

FORTIFY YOUR BODY WITH PLANT-BASED IRON

One of the first actions I took when I decided to become healthy was to undergo several tests to understand more about my body and what it needed. Surprisingly it turned out I was taking in too much iron. Yes, too much. Too much iron can lead to serious health issues, such as liver disease, hypothyroidism, certain cancers, arthritis, and heart disease. This is not to say that iron isn't good for you—we need moderate amounts of it for countless reasons, especially for your hemoglobin, which transports oxygen in the blood.

Too little iron and you'll experience fatigue. The problem is that animal foods are very high in heme iron, which absorbs very easily into your body. If you eat meat regularly, chances are you are receiving more iron than your body can handle. Plants, on the other hand, are rich in nonheme iron, which our bodies have an easier time regulating. It's found in everything from dark leafy greens to beans and legumes, from whole grains to nuts and seeds. When you eat plants, you'll only be receiving a moderate, healthy amount of iron that won't overload your body.

Plant Foods with Lots of Iron

- Vegetables: Swiss chard, collard greens, spinach, mushrooms
- Nuts and Seeds: almonds, cashews, pistachios, hemp, pumpkin, sunflower
- Legumes: black beans, chickpeas, lentils, soybeans, tofu, tempeh
- Grains: amaranth, brown rice, oats, quinoa, spelt
- Fruits: dried apricots, prune juice

SHOPPING

SHOP SMART AND SAVE MONEY

I was never the shopper in my household before going whole food, plant based. My better half, Tracey, did most of it. Now I am indeed the shopper. A shopping beast, in fact. I go to farmers' markets, to big stores, to bodegas, to health-food shops, to street fairs. I love it.

I particularly enjoy finding new stores with unfamiliar cuisines. These places were once as foreign to me as the countries that make the products they sell, but now I understand the power of these different and unusual fruits and vegetables (see pages 67–70). For example, breadfruit: Everyone knows what bread is, everyone knows what fruit is, but something called *breadfruit?* Now I know it and love it!

Most of us shop by beelining to the processed food aisles, where we find our cereals, cheeses, mixes, and so forth. Not healthy! These aisles are no longer included in my journey. I spend all my time in the produce aisles now.

The best place to start shopping for healthy foods is to march right over to the fruits and veggies. Start each week by introducing yourself to a new vegetable. Do research on how to cook that vegetable to best maintain its nutrients. Take kale, for example. Find it in your market. Buy it. Bring it home. Study the best ways to cook it. In other words, learn your food.

Then, graduate to another fruit or vegetable. That's how you get a solid understanding of your food repertoire. Next, travel over to the spice aisle and find new and exotic spices (see page 104).

Avoid the processed food aisle at all cost. Make this your mantra: I will not eat junk food. I will not eat packaged food. I will not eat ingredients I can't pronounce. Steer clear of the snack food section. These foods are just empty calories. Instead, indulge with figs and raisins, bananas and apples. You can still have sweets. You just don't have to eat ones that damage your health. One good tip is to not shop when you're hungry. You're liable to disregard all this advice and go for the tastiest, fastest foods you can find.

If you're in a store that doesn't have a wide selection of unprocessed foods, work hard to find something good. It's there. Maybe it's an apple or a banana. Maybe it's boxed raisins. If this is your local store, let yourself be known. Encourage the staff to bring in better foods. They may think there's no demand for these foods, but you will prove them wrong.

I am quite lucky to live near several farmers' markets, where I buy most of my produce. If you are equally fortunate, you may have these markets near you. Seek them out and buy from them. You'll be getting healthy foods, and the markets will sense a greater demand for their crops and bring in more produce.

Can't shop at a farmers' market? Even in food swamps—places with only unhealthy food options—you may still find an oasis in the frozen section. It's true that the closest thing you'll find to fresh produce in most bodegas is a sad basket of bananas, but frozen fruits and vegetables offer nearly the same nutritional bang for your buck as their fresh counterparts. That's because they are frozen almost immediately after they are picked, so their vitamins, minerals, antioxidants, and phytonutrients stay preserved for months. Frozen produce also tends to be cheaper.

I still encourage people to do a canvas of their neighborhood and see which stores carry which fresh foods as it's good to support local businesses and farmers. These fresh food oases exist. You just have to find them. Even in the most desolate areas there is smart, fresh food.

Here's something you may not realize: the cost of eating healthy is less than eating nonhealthy. Why? Because the basics of a vegan diet are inexpensive. Rice. Beans. Chickpeas. Potatoes. Carrots. Onions. Garlic. Oatmeal. Apples. Oranges. Peanut butter. Whole-grain bread. We're not talking fancy steak and expensive cheeses. We're talking basic foods that make sense, make you healthy, and don't make you broke.

There are a few more ways to save even more money:

- Buy in bulk, particularly different kinds of dried beans. These are your go-to foods, and they are very cheap. One bag of lentils that can last you a whole week costs about $2. Think of all you can make: lentil burgers, lentil soups, lentil casseroles, and more.

- Rely on vegetables for your main courses. They are wonderfully inexpensive. A head of kale can last two or three days, and it can be mixed into so many meals. A head of celery costs about $2 and will last you the whole week. Tomatoes are delicious, go with everything, and are inexpensive. You get the best prices when vegetables are in season, so do a little research and plan accordingly.

- Find other places to buy foods, and indulge in some comparison shopping. Buy from farmers' markets, join a local co-op, create a co-op on your own if you're entrepreneurial, or see if your church or other organization can sponsor a food co-op to purchase in bulk. The goal is to create a community of enough local buyers to create a continuing market for healthy foods.

If you start out with the mind-set that eating healthy is less expensive than eating junk, the odds are excellent it will become so.

LEARN HOW TO READ FOOD LABELS

Reading food labels is one of the most important parts of your health journey. That label tells you almost everything you need to know about the product's contents, from its salt to its sugar, from its carbs to its fat, and so on. And yes, these are things you *need* to know. To truly read a label well, you'll want to become a nutritional detective. Ingredients and numbers can be misleading. Don't be fooled by foggy claims and confusing information.

Start by investigating one topic at a time. In my case I first looked into sodium (salt), which can contribute to high blood pressure and heart disease if consumed in large amounts. I studied all the different ways that sodium can be hidden on a label, such as sea salt, fleur de sel, or monosodium glutamate, until I mastered all these various salt disguises and could tell quickly if a product contained too much. Often if you just look for the word "salt," you won't actually see all the salt inside the product—you'll only see as much as the food company hopes you'll see.

Then I moved on to sugar. I learned about the ways sugar is sneakily added to foods, usually in forms like high-fructose syrup, grape juice, rice bran syrup, molasses, lactose, glucose, and others. Like salt, sugar can be called many different things, but it's still sugar.

Next I studied grains, multigrains, and all the different ways packages use slogans like "made with whole grains," which might mean just a tiny amount of whole grains inside. If the product doesn't have a good amount of fiber, or whole grains aren't among the first ingredients, there's likely to be few whole grains in the food.

How to Tell if Bread Is Healthy

Walk into the bread aisle and you'll see dozens and dozens of products. It's overwhelming. Some of the bread is brown—that means it's healthy, right? Many say things like "multigrain." The truth is, most of that is marketing mumbo jumbo.

In truth, all bread is processed. After all, there isn't a bread tree. You have to take dough, culture it with yeast, and bake it in an oven. The best and healthiest bread has as few chemicals added as possible. Here's a trick I learned: Check out the fiber content in grams on the nutrition label. Now multiply that number by 6. Is it more than the total number of carbohydrates in the bread per serving? If not, you should avoid that bread.

For example, take Arnold 100% Whole Wheat Bread. That sounds healthy, right? Well, the label says it has 3 grams of fiber and 19 grams of carbohydrates per serving. Multiply those 3 grams of fiber by 6 and you get 18, which is less than the 19 grams of carbs. Not healthy. Now check out Ezekiel 4:9 Sprouted Whole Grain Bread. It also has 3 grams of fiber, but just 15 grams of carbs per serving. If you multiply the 3 grams of fiber by 6 you get 18—more than the 15 grams of carbs. Healthy!

You always want to check out how much fat is in every food. Again, you might be surprised to see there's much more than you might have thought. Try to avoid eating any saturated fat, unless you're eating whole plants like avocados and nuts.

Remember that the ingredients are listed in the order of how much is in the product by weight. The first three or so tend to make up most of the food. If these are mostly oils or sugars, you don't want that food.

Also important: Learn about the serving size. This will help you determine how much fat, calories, salt, and so on are truly inside the product. Say it's a can of noodles that you think would make a nice dinner, but upon careful examination you see the can actually contains three servings, so you'd have to multiply all the numbers pertaining to salt, sugar, and fat by three if you eat the contents of the whole can—and those numbers can really add up.

The Daily Value will tell you how many required vitamins and minerals are in the product. In general, if the food has 5 percent or less of a nutrient per serving, it is not considered a high source of it. You want at least 15 percent for that food to be considered valuable for that nutrient.

The best part of a whole-food, plant-based diet is that you don't have to worry about labels when you're buying fresh veggies and fruits! When did you ever see an avocado with an ingredient list? On an apple, the only label you'll find is the number sequence to see if the apple is organic or uses a high level of pesticide (which is a good thing to know about). Briefly, a four-digit code starting with the number 4 or 5 means that the fruit was conventionally raised, and a five-digit code starting with the number 8 means that it has been genetically modified. A five-digit number starting with a 9 means the item is organic.

Be sure to watch out for misleading claims. The word "light" sounds healthy, but it's almost meaningless, and often just refers to a product that has been watered down to reduce calories. "Light" doesn't mean healthy. Likewise, "all natural" is meaningless; it simply says that there is one or more natural food within the product. "Fruit-flavored" may sound healthy, but all it implies is that some kind of natural fruit flavoring has been used in the product—it still may well be fruit free.

Keep it simple and stick to whole foods that have one, and only one, ingredient.

Organic Foods

Should you shop for organic foods? They are indeed the ideal choice, but they aren't always the best choice. For folks on a strict budget, organic foods can be prohibitively expensive. Don't ever think you are a bad mom or dad because you aren't buying organic produce for your kids. Your basic supermarket fruits and vegetables are perfectly fine. They may have more pesticide residue compared to organic, though, so you should wash them extensively before cooking. (The easiest way is to soak them in salty water for 20 minutes.)

Unfortunately the term "organic" can mean many different things in different places. Recommendation: If you really want to evolve into the organic area, look into Dr. Michael Greger's video "Are Organic Foods Healthier?" for a good primer on the topic.

MAKE YOUR KITCHEN A SMART KITCHEN

Just as you are now learning about different foods to eat on your health journey, you should start looking into appropriate cooking utensils. The more you learn about how to cook healthy, the more you will learn about what to cook with. And the more you become versed in nutrient-dense foods, the more you will want to make sure you keep them as healthy as possible throughout the cooking process.

As for me, I never even owned a mixer because I never mixed anything. I never had a food processor. Now I have both.

Consider investing in a hot-air fryer, which is an excellent way to prepare fried soul-food classics (with a vegan twist) without greasy, unhealthy oils. Likewise, an electric pressure cooker can cook your beans and prepare delicious meals that you can then freeze and store for days.

For the more experienced cooks out there, a spiralizer is an inexpensive tool that will help you turn fresh vegetables into veggie noodles. It looks like a large pencil sharpener and it works easily: you put in the vegetables and out come spirals that you can cook.

Colanders are necessary to drain the water off all the vegetables you'll be buying (and the whole-wheat pasta you'll be cooking as well).

Think about buying a good fresh-herb keeper. The more you discover the goodness of herbs, the more you'll want to keep them around. Also useful, and very inexpensive, is a garlic peeler, which makes removing the sticky skin a snap.

Do you have a good set of knives? You'll need them to chop, mince, and dice all your favorite vegetables down to size.

A mandolin is another excellent tool for cutting your vegetables to the right cooking portion; just be careful you don't cut yourself on its sharp blades (although if you do, you'll be like every other cook at some point or another). I always keep bandages handy.

You'll want a steamer basket to steam your vegetables evenly and perfectly (because you're no longer frying them in oils).

A little more expensive, but totally worth the price, is a two-speed hand blender so you can mix up beverages and sauces right in the pan. Another of the best tools you can buy is one of the cheapest: for just a few dollars you can get a good salad spinner that will dry your lettuce in seconds.

If you like desserts, consider purchasing a Yonanas, a frozen dessert maker that creates delicious banana-based ice cream. And speaking of fruit, if you don't have a corer, you can pick one up for less than $10, and it will make it so much easier to cook up your apples or other fruits. And a citrus juicer is also a great way to get all the juices out of your oranges and other fruits.

I also had to buy new bowls because now I eat enormous salads. My old bowls were only a fraction of what I needed. Tracey and I also needed new storage containers because we so often make dinners that are also the next day's lunch.

EAT THE SPICES OF LIFE

Before I was healthy, spices meant salt and pepper. If I was feeling like an Iron Chef, maybe some cinnamon. That was it.

Nowadays, however, I have dozens of strange and exotic spices on my wall. Even if you already know how much better spices can make food, you might not be aware of their nutritional benefits.

Every week I discover a new spice: where it came from, what makes it healthy, and how to cook with it.

Herbs and Spices

Have you ever wondered what the difference is between herbs and spices, but were too embarrassed to ask? Don't worry, you're not alone. I had no idea until I began eating plant based.

The difference comes down to which part of the plant is used. If it's the plant's leaf, it's an herb. If it's another part, such as dried seeds, roots, or bark, then it's a spice. Both are incredibly healthy, and both are delicious!

The first herb I studied was basil. It may not sound very exotic or fun, but basil not only helps make a great pesto and other sauces, it has medicinal benefits, such as helping to suppress coughs and colds.

Next came the spice cinnamon (the Ceylon variety is the best of the lot), which most people already know has many uses in cooking. But cinnamon also can lower your blood sugar, which was very important to me when I had diabetes. Cinnamon is also filled with antioxidants and has anti-inflammatory properties as well. Cumin was next. It's another spice that can help manage your blood sugar levels, and it goes great with my favorite beans and grains.

Then came garlic, which I learned is underused and underappreciated. Yes, it can give you bad breath, but it also gives you a good life. You can eat it so many ways. Store it in a mesh bag at room temperature (you can also store it in the crisper drawer of your refrigerator) and it'll keep for a few weeks, and you'll sometimes even see stems growing from them, a real indicator that food is alive. Put peeled garlic in your blender and mix it into soups or add it to salad dressings and stews. Its uses are endless and so are its health benefits, including lowering blood sugar and cholesterol levels, and it may even help prevent the common cold. Why not take garlic rather than medicine? No side effects, great taste! (Just gargle some mouthwash before that hot date!)

Next up is ginger, which is superb for your digestion, helps with your absorption of nutrients, and is anti-inflammatory. It can even help soothe sore muscles. Ginger works well in baked goods and desserts, but is also useful in sauces and stir fries, among many other uses.

You must learn about turmeric (and its active ingredient, curcumin), another anti-inflammatory spice that also lowers your blood sugar level, may lower your risk of heart disease, and ward off cancer. It's even been shown to help people suffering from cognitive decline. Turmeric is best when mixed with black pepper (which dramatically increases the absorption of curcumin and its health benefits in the body), and you can add it to salad dressings, curries, vegetables, and soups. I also love to sprinkle it along with some nutritional yeast on my popcorn.

These are just a few of the dozens of spices that you'll eventually grow to love, both for their flavor and their health benefits. Something to keep in mind: you'll need a spice rack. Maybe two, because you'll keep learning about new spices. You'll become something of a modern day Magellan, traveling to different spice shops and filling your home with new and exotic spices from around the world.

DINE OUT SMART

One of the biggest errors people make when they go vegan is to think that the only place they can get a plant-based meal is a plant-based restaurant.

Actually, you can get a terrific vegan meal at almost any restaurant. You just have to order smart.

First, the appetizers. Here is where most restaurants show off their vegetables and small dishes. You can easily make a wonderful meal out of two appetizers, feel full and content, and never go near anything that came from an animal.

Next consider the side dishes. Most restaurants have plates of vegetables that you can ask to be prepared without butter, such as broccoli, mushrooms, string beans, and kale. Combine these with an appetizer and you have an excellent healthy meal. If you don't see sides listed specifically, then look for what comes with the steaks or the chops. If there's a pot roast and broccoli dish, then you know the kitchen has broccoli. Just skip the roast.

You can also just try asking for what you want. Tell the waiter you'd like asparagus, chopped up with mushroom, kale, and red onions; you'll have a great meal made from the foods you've spotted on the menu. Restaurants these days are used to catering to dietary restrictions, and most waiters won't bat an eye when you order off the menu. If they won't let you order this way, politely explain that you aren't able to eat anything on the menu with meat or dairy, and if they could recommend a solution. More times than not, a chef will find a way to accommodate you.

Fast food is another issue. It's not likely to be healthy, but most of these places have at least a salad. Just be careful of the dressing. A healthy bed of greens can easily become a nutritional nightmare by bathing them in Thousand Island dressing. These days many fast food places have started serving vegan burgers, such as the Impossible Whopper at Burger King. Remember, it's not health food. An Impossible Whopper is almost as bad for you as a regular Whopper. But it's better than nothing, and at the very least you are saving animals and the environment. I myself prefer vegetables to fake meats, but if you're on a road trip or otherwise in a pinch, the occasional plant-based burger indulgence is perfectly fine.

Go Plant Based for the Environment

In this book we're focusing on the health reasons you should give up meat and go plant based, but that isn't the only reason. By helping your health, you are also helping the health of the planet. Here are only a few reasons why:

- If every American removed a single serving of chicken from their diet, it would be the equivalent of removing half a million cars from the road.

- By going vegan the average American reduces the country's carbon emissions by 1.5 tons per year.

- Cows, pigs, chickens, and turkeys are the largest producers of methane in the United States—a greenhouse gas that is 20 times more effective at trapping heat than carbon dioxide.

- One calorie from animal protein requires 11 times as much fossil fuel energy compared to plant protein, and all told, eating a meat-based diet creates 7 times more greenhouse gas emissions than a vegan diet.

- Almost half of all the fresh water used in the United States goes to raising animals for food.

- It takes more than 2,400 gallons of water to create just a single pound of meat. By not eating that pound, you'd save the water equivalent of not showering for six months.

- Animals raised for meat and dairy create almost 90,000 pounds of excrement per second, much of which contaminates ground water.

- Thirty percent of the world's entire land mass is devoted to grazing animals for slaughter—a space larger than the surface area of the moon.

- Every minute the equivalent of seven football fields are bulldozed just to create space for farmed animals.

MOVE YOUR BODY

REDEFINE THE WORD *EXERCISE*

Exercise is an important part of your new health plan. But remember, exercise is not a gym membership. It's a not a spin bike or a hot-yoga studio. Exercise is simply movement. The best way to exercise for health is to build as much movement into your life as you can.

Every day we have choices between activity or inactivity. Do you take an escalator, or do you take the stairs? Do you walk a few blocks, or do you take a bus? Do you sit all day at your desk, or do you get up and walk around every half an hour?

Being sedentary is the enemy of health just as much as processed junk food is. Movement is crucial for your blood circulation. It increases your brain size. It prevents memory loss. It boosts your mood. It reduces depression. Studies have shown that movement helps us feel better, both physically and emotionally. Avoiding exercise can increase the chance of back pain, high cholesterol, organ damage, bad posture, insomnia, muscle degeneration, and many other conditions.

Although there is no hard-and-fast rule, in general the World Health Organization recommends adults aged 18 to 64 should get at least 150 minutes of moderate-intensity aerobic physical activity each week, or at least 75 minutes of vigorous-intensity aerobic physical activity throughout the week, along with some kind of muscle strengthening movement for all major muscle groups at least twice a week. Don't worry, this sounds a lot more difficult than it actually is. I barely have any free time during my week, yet I still manage to squeeze in exercise. I'll show you my best tactics in the following sections.

TAKE THE STAIRS (AND OTHER DAILY TIPS)

There are many, many ways you can add movement to your life. The following are just a few. If you want more, be inventive. Find ways to move that you never thought possible. Your body will thank you.

First off, stop sitting. Sitting is the new smoking. During the 1950s, a Scottish epidemiologist named Jerry Morris devised a curious study: He followed the health of London bus drivers and conductors. All the variables—age, social class, diet—were the same except for one: the conductors were constantly on their feet collecting tickets and ascending and descending up to 750 steps daily on double-decker buses, while the drivers were constantly sitting. By the end of the study, Morris found that the conductors were half as likely to suffer heart attacks compared to the drivers.

Are bus drivers genetically more likely to have a heart attack compared to ticket collectors? Of course not. But bus drivers are more likely to be sitting all day, which decreases circulation, causes blood to pool in your feet, and promotes obesity. If you're sitting all day, then you have the same risk of heart disease as the bus drivers.

Many Americans sit at a computer for work. I'm not going to say everyone should quit their jobs and work construction, but there are simple ways to be more active while staying productive. A standing desk at your office or home can help you stretch and move. These desks aren't very expensive, particularly if you do what I do and use a small metal music stand desk. Don't only stand while you're at your office; stand as much as you can, at meetings, on the bus, at parties. I used to do the New York subway dash for a seat on the train, but now I think the lucky ones are those of us who stand instead of sit.

Likewise, use the stairs as much as you can, even if you work or live on a high floor. You can always climb, say, halfway and then take the elevator if you get tired. The better shape you get into, the more you can walk. Buy yourself a small barbell set to use at home. They don't have to be heavy. Use them to build strength and to get your heart rate up. Do jumping jacks whenever you can—after getting up in the morning, between meetings, whenever you can do them without feeling self-conscious. People won't think you're silly for exercising during the day. They'll be jealous.

Don't think of your lunch hour as simply a time to eat. It's a great opportunity to take a long walk, trot up and down some stairs, or at least roam the corridors. Take the long way to the bathroom or the printer. Walk to your co-worker's desk for a chat instead of calling or instant messaging. Walking meetings are becoming increasingly common. Instead of having everyone sit in a chair for hours, consider walking and talking at the same time. Maybe you're lucky enough to have an assistant, but don't always delegate your work. Get up whenever you can to find or file your papers. And forget about happy hours. Try some exercise hours. After work, get a group of people together who'd rather talk and walk in some scenery.

Housework can actually be good exercise, and fun. Don't rely on a robotic vacuum cleaner when you can push around a vacuum or a broom and get your heartrate up. If you have a yard, think about pushing a mower over your grass instead of turning on an electric one. Even making your bed every morning can get your body moving and your heart pumping.

When it's time to stream your shows, do it while walking on an exercise machine, be it a bike or a treadmill. Or take it a step further and do a little jump roping. It's good for your heart and costs almost nothing.

Walking a dog is a great way to get some exercise and make your four-legged friend happy. I even know a few people who've trained their cats to go outside on a leash. (Note: Not that many cats will do this. But if you've got one who will, not only will you get some exercise, you'll be the talk of your town.)

Install a pull-up bar in your house. A few pull-ups a day will improve your posture and strengthen your arms and core.

Studies have shown that someone who does these exercises is just as fit as someone who goes to the gym. There's even a fascinating study showing that a cleaning staff who were consciously told that they were exercising were healthier than the ones who did not realize they were exercising. Simply by telling employees that their daily work involved serious exercise, Harvard psychologists were apparently able to lower the cleaning staff's blood pressure, shave pounds off their bodies, and improve their body fat and waist-to-hip ratios. Self-awareness, it seems, was as important a factor as the actual exercise.

In other words, your mind and your body are connected. Your intent assists you in the goals you are trying to reach. Tell yourself you're going to move. Insist you are being active when you are, even if it's just taking the long way to the subway.

It's about movement, not about a gym membership.

BREATHE

Part of staying well—and exercising well—is breathing well. Yes, everyone breathes, and we don't stop until we die. But that doesn't mean we do it well. Most people pay little attention to their breath, not realizing that they may be taking in too little oxygen or refraining from taking those long, deep breaths that ground us.

The power of breath is important all around the world. And although we breathe every day, in our culture we are never formally taught how to breathe best for health, despite its vital role in moving oxygen to the brain, in helping your heart beat, in managing stress. And yet you don't hear about it in schools, at our places of worship, or even at our doctor's office.

In the yogic tradition, the breath is the very foundation of life. It connects the body with the spirit. Many Eastern-based exercises, such as tai chi, are based on breathing practices that improve the body's use of energy as well as improve posture and strengthen your diaphragm muscles.

Good breathing should be part of your exercise program too. Breathing well increases your blood flow throughout your body, and can prevent injuries, such as hernias and back pain, and prevent spikes in blood pressure that harm blood vessels.

I like to practice the 8–4–2 regimen. Every day I take eight deep breaths, four quick breaths, and then two deep breaths held for a long time. Then I breathe in as much as I can, for as long as I can, and then I breathe out. I do that three times.

There are plenty of other such methods, including Dr. Andrew Weil's (author of *Spontaneous Healing*), who recommends a 4–7–8 method:

- Exhale completely through your mouth, making a whoosh sound.

- Close your mouth and inhale quietly through your nose to a mental count of four.

- Hold your breath for a count of seven.

- Exhale completely through your mouth, making a whoosh sound to a count of eight.

- This is one breath. Now inhale again and repeat the cycle three more times for a total of four breaths.

There are many other methods. Search breathing exercises on the web and you'll find one that suits you. You'll be amazed at how much better you'll feel.

KEEPING
IT GOING

FIND A SPIRITUAL PRACTICE

"There is no greater force for change than when a community discovers what it cares about."—Margaret Wheatley

Food is complicated. It isn't simply what we put in our mouths. Food actually becomes a large part of how we see ourselves—as carnivores, omnivores, or herbivores. It even conjures up memories from childhood, from sharing a hot dog with Dad at a ballgame to eating at the local fast-food joint with your friends, from enjoying your grandmother's famous casserole to the pint of ice cream you turn to when you're sad. Unfortunately, for the most part, these are foods that aggravate and cause disease. For some people it can be difficult to overcome years of habits and memories.

Success isn't just a matter of saying, "I won't eat that stuff again." Few people are that willful. You will want support. Part of that comes from your doctor, your friends, and your family, but I believe that another part of the strength that pushes you forward is spirituality. You have to look inward to build the emotional strength it takes to reverse a lifetime of unhealthy foods.

When I say spiritual, I don't necessarily mean church on Sundays or temple on Saturdays. Spirituality can be religious, but it can also be nonreligious, such as a meditation practice, yoga, painting, or anything else that centers your inner strength. With it, instead of picking up that double cheeseburger and a soda, you pick up a paintbrush or a yoga mat, if that's where you find your relaxation.

As for me, I am a Christian, and I grew up in a Christian household. At the same time, I don't shy away from the power of all belief systems. I enjoy reading the Koran and the Torah and other religious texts because I believe they share a universal foundation that guides us to discovering our better selves. Too often we don't equate our better selves with what we eat or consider that our bodies are a gift from the Creator and we should not abuse that gift.

I believe that being spiritual means finding ways to center yourself. Humans are in a constant state of imbalance, and to many people, bad food has become their outlet and refuge. Because it can feel momentarily relaxing, you might binge on a pint of Chunky Monkey ice cream and think you have calmed yourself down. In reality, the opposite has happened: You have upset your system, you have given it unhealthy food, you have raised your cholesterol levels, you have added unneeded weight, and you have taken another step down the path to chronic disease and chronic pain. You might feel good for a moment, but you will feel worse later. Trust me.

I won't pretend that changing your diet isn't stressful. Often, you will need an outlet. You need something that gives you the strength you once thought unhealthy food provided.

When I am stressed out and consider eating something harmful, I take a moment to sit down, reflect on my feelings, pause, and try a small moment of meditation. Other times, I listen to music. I also like to pick up a positive quote, one that inspires me to understand the importance of eating healthy. Reading a quote, like the ones in this section, can be very centering.

"In every crisis there is a message. Crises are nature's way of forcing change—breaking down old structures, shaking loose negative habits so that something new and better can take their place."—Susan Taylor

NEVER BEAT YOURSELF UP

"The pessimist sees difficulty in every opportunity. The optimist sees opportunity in every difficulty."
—Winston Churchill

There are going to be good days, there are going to be great days, but there are also going to be hard days when you make mistakes. Maybe you couldn't help yourself and you scarfed down a bag of chocolate chip cookies. Maybe you devoured an enormous bowl of pasta with cream sauce. Maybe you even ate a bacon cheeseburger. Don't fret. Everyone slips up now and then. This is a lifelong journey. You have time to get it right.

When I first started my health journey, there were several moments when my appetite got the best of me and I gulped down a nice big piece of cake. It didn't happen too often; it happened less and less as the months passed, and I never became angry at myself. You shouldn't either. No one has perfect willpower. Remember that a bend in the road is not the end of the road unless you fail to make the turn.

It's not what you do one day, it's what you do *every* day. Forgive yourself, laugh, and move on. Learn from your mistakes and think of strategies for avoiding them next time. Your mind and body will evolve to the next level.

"You always pass failure on your way to success."
—Mickey Rooney

ASK FOR HELP

"Never bend your head. Always hold it high. Look the world straight in the eye."—Helen Keller

You are not alone. In fact, you would be amazed at how many good people are in this whole-food, plant-based space, people who very much want others to ask them about their health and their diet. You can't imagine what an excited and devoted group it is. They want to share this information and they will do so, kindly and with patience, when you ask.

But the key is to ask. If you don't, then you won't hear what these wonderful people have to say.

Information about a whole-food, plant-based diet can be found everywhere. You can spot it in online newsletters, blogs, magazines, and journals. You can join meet-up groups, find support groups, or attend lectures. If you live in New York, we host events every three months at Brooklyn Borough Hall. And remember, whenever you find an expert you'd like to talk to, e-mail, reach out on social media, or pick up the phone. No matter how busy people are, they welcome newcomers to the journey.

As we all learned in the third grade, no question is a dumb question. Whatever you need to know is important to you, and therefore it's important.

"A sure way for one to lift himself up is by helping to lift someone else."—Booker T. Washington

PROCEED AT YOUR OWN PACE

"A champion is defined not by their wins, but by how they can recover when they fall."—Serena Williams

Your journey is unique. Don't look at other people and think you're falling behind or that you're far ahead. You are where only you can be. You may be participating in meatless Mondays, you might be going meatless once a month, you might be all meatless. That's up to you, and it's your business and only yours. You will eventually get to the best place you can. Just make sure you keep moving. Procrastination cannot become stagnation.

We all wind up in different places. I myself am oil free, but not everyone is. If you're not, then find the healthiest oil you can use. Maybe you'll eventually decide you don't want oil. Terrific! But then is then and now is now. Some people don't like beans. That's fine, but find a good alternative. Some people are gluten free. Discover foods that allow you to be healthy without gluten. (Hint: try quinoa.) It's your decision!

It's all about your pace. But the mere fact that you have a pace means you have movement, and movement is good. Pace yourself well, and you will be well.

"It is time for every one of us to roll up our sleeves and put ourselves at the top of our commitment list."
—Marian Wright Edelman

WATCH YOUR WEIGHT (DROP)

"It is not true that people stop pursuing their dreams because they grow old; they grow old because they stop pursuing their dreams."—Gabriel García Márquez

Here's the good news. Just about everyone who switches to a whole-food, plant-based diet loses weight. This means you probably will too. And you'll do it by eating as much as you want of the best foods Mother Nature has to offer. You won't be eating high-calorie processed foods. You won't be eating nutritionally light foods. You won't be eating sugary, salty snacks. You won't even have to worry about counting your calories because all your whole-food, plant-based foods will be low in calories and high in goodness and fiber.

Because these foods are so healthy, you will find that you'll fill up faster and stay full longer than ever before. My breakfast smoothie keeps me going for four hours. By the time I finish lunch, I am full pretty much until dinner time. I didn't even realize how much less I was eating.

Eventually I lost 35 pounds even though I wasn't especially trying to lose weight. I was just trying to take control of my diabetes. Tracey and I looked at photos taken of us on vacation in 2016 . . . and needless to say, we don't leave them out for people to see. Our bodies have transformed so much we barely recognize our former selves.

That said, it's not a good idea to eat only for weight loss. For some, weight loss is merely for vanity's sake. If all you're interested in is looking good, you're not paying attention to nutrition. You might even end up trying one of those silly diets where you just eat steaks or you down lots of juices. These gimmicks may help you lose weight momentarily, but that weight loss doesn't last. And you're hurting your body in the process.

However, when you eat a whole-food, plant-based diet, you are changing your lifestyle, not just what's on your dinner plate. So not only are you on the road to great health, you keep the weight off for good because you always feel full, happy, and content with your food. No wishing you could eat that chocolate fudge every night, no pining for thick milkshakes while at work, no dreaming of a huge egg-and-sausage sandwich in the morning.

Ok, I lied to you earlier in the book. There *is* one expensive part about going plant based. Your wardrobe! You may have to buy new clothes to fit your healthy new body. I stubbornly wore my old clothes for so long that people thought I was seriously ill. I went from a 36-inch to a 32-inch waist. (I keep one pair of large pants as a reminder of what I used to look like. The rest I donated to charity.) One friend who went healthy last year dropped down from a 52-inch waist to a 38. He sent me a photo showing how he can now stand in just one leg of his old pants.

Think about it: inside your body right now is a healthy one just waiting to emerge. Now go and find it!

"I'm a success today because I had a friend who believed in me and I didn't have the heart to let him down."
—Abraham Lincoln

DON'T BRAG (WHEN YOU START LOOKING OH SO GOOD)

"It's been said that no one can really motivate anyone else; all you can do is instill a positive attitude and hope it catches on."—Eddie Robinson

You might become annoying when you realize how wonderful you look and feel. Inside that unhealthy body is a prisoner, so when you are paroled and start to enjoy what freedom really is, you may want to let everyone else share that freedom with you.

Be careful. You have to meet people where they are. You can't push them past what they can do. Maybe they want to get healthy just as badly as you, but they're not ready to go plant based. They're not ready to give up their old soul-food favorites. When they are, they'll come to you and ask for help. In the meantime, just keep your enjoyment of your new body and your excellent health to yourself. (Others will see anyway!)

"The power for creating a better future is contained in the present moment: You create a good future by creating a good present."—Eckhart Tolle

HAVE FUN!

"Things work out best for those who make the best of how things work out."—John Wooden

I can't think of anything more important than having fun while you're making a big lifestyle change. Why? Because if you consider all this as just a job, something you don't really want to do but feel you must, then you won't stick with it. You will burn out.

Don't think of this as work! There are so many ways you can experience fun while experiencing health. Experiment with new foods and discover all kinds of tastes that make you happy. Find spices that make your meals taste better than you ever imagined. Eat out smart at restaurants and experience the wonderful sense of feeling full, but not stuffed. Try all kinds of new exercises that you didn't realize were so good for you, like climbing stairs instead of taking the elevator or walking to the store instead of driving. Search out new places to eat and new places to shop.

In other words, enjoy yourself! If you can, get your other half involved—or your best friend or sibling. That can be part of the fun too. You can work together and make it a game. Who can find the best new foods? Who can cook the best new meals? Who takes the most steps in a day? Who can lower their cholesterol the most in three months? Who can cure their diabetes first?

Learn to cook healthy meals and invite friends over. Show people that you still love food. In fact you love it more than ever because now you know it's not just about how it tastes; it's how it makes you feel.

And you *will* feel great!

"I don't like short-term solutions; they can come back and bite you in the behind later."—Caroline R. Jones

GET IN TOUCH WITH ME

Now that you've read all my steps for a healthy life, think them all over. If you have any questions, e-mail me. Connect with my office on social media. Talk to me. Come to my lectures. I am here to help you. I really am.

"How far you go in life depends on your being tender with the young, compassionate with the aged, sympathetic with the striving and tolerant of the weak and strong. Because someday in your life you will have been all of these."
—George Washington Carver

CHAPTER 4

RECIPES

Breakfast

Power Red Smoothie—Queen Afua

Purple Sweet Potato Smoothie—Dr. Michael Greger

Lemon-Infused Quinoa Breakfast Bowl—Rip Esselstyn

Overnight Chia Oats with Berries—Michelle McMacken

Powerhouse Oats—Caldwell Esselstyn

Chickpea Omelet—Charity Morgan

Airport Oatmeal—Moby

Appetizers and Snacks

Spicy Thai Meatballs with Orange-Chili Dipping Sauce—Del Sroufe

Sweet Potato Cornbread—Zakiyaa Michèl

Sriracha–Almond Butter Hummus—Robin Robertson

Stuffed Grape Leaves—Marco Borges

Black Bean–Pumpkin Quesadillas with Sweet Pepper Salsa and
Lime Crema—Andrea Nordby

Maple-Jerk Hummus—CC Péan

Soups

Jackfruit and Okra Gumbo—Darshana Thacker

Blooming Black Bean Soup—Queen Afua

Creamy Tomato Basil Bisque—Del Sroufe

Bad Ass Vegan Sweet Potato Soup—John Lewis

Cream of Zucchini-Kale Soup—Nina Curtis

Pepper-Pot Soup—Raymond Jackson

Vegetable Soup—Dorothy Adams

Thai Sweet Potato Soup—Ayinde Howell

Salads

Caesar Salad with Suzy's Caesar Dressing—Suzy Amis Cameron

Super Green Live Salad and Avocado Dressing—Queen Afua

Roasted Beet and Potato Salad—Jenné Claiborne

Eat What Elephants Eat Bowl—Dominick Thompson

Taco Salad—Taymer Mason

Main Dishes

Oven-Roasted Moroccan Squash with Tahini Sauce—CC Péan

Hoppin' John Stew—Darshana Thacker

Sweet Potato Enchiladas with Cashew-Chili Sour Cream—Chad Sarno and Derek Sarno

Pasta with Kale and Sausage—Donna Green-Goodman

Polenta Stacks with Black Bean and Corn Salsa—Robin Robertson

Roasted Veggie Lasagna—Dotsie Bausch

Chipotle Mac 'n' Cheese—Megan Sadd

Quinoa and Tempeh Stir-Fry with Broccoli and Carrots—Gregory Brown

Forest Bowls with Earthy Vegetables and Turmeric Cashew Sauce—Andrea Nordby

Black Bean Tacos—Paul McCartney

Greens and Beans—Tracey Collins

Stovies—Alan Cumming

Sweet Potato–Collard Green Saag Paneer—Raymond Jackson

Spicy Quinoa Meatballs—Yvonne Ardestani

Hawaiian Sloppy Jacks—Angela Means

Grits and Greens—Robin Robertson

Pasta with Charred Tomatoes and White Wine Sauce—Leslie Durso

African Greens Mélange—CC Péan

B.Y. Burgers—B.Y. Jennings

Desserts

Three-Ingredient Ice Cream—Eric Adams

Basmati Rice Pudding—Dr. Fiona B. Lewis

No-Bake Sweet Potato Bars with Raw Gingerbread Crust—Jenné Claiborne

Easy Chocolate Truffles—Robin Robertson

Chewy Peanut Butter Cookies—Charity Morgan

Fruit Pizza—Donna Green-Goodman

BREAKFAST

POWER RED SMOOTHIE

International best-selling author **Queen Afua** *is a certified holistic health practitioner, devoted wellness advocate, and influential global consultant with over 40 years of experience.*

Makes 2 to 4 servings

"No need to add any sugar to this smoothie, as the fruits provide sufficient sweetness. The mixture can also be poured into ice pop molds or ice cube trays and put into the freezer. Serve later as a delicious, nutritious frozen treat."

3 to 4 red apples	½ cup raspberries
½ cup blueberries	2 small bananas
½ cup blackberries	

Wash, core, and cut the apples. Put the apple pieces into a high-speed blender or food processor and blend until smooth. Add the berries and bananas and blend until smooth. Pour into glasses or mugs and serve.

PURPLE SWEET POTATO SMOOTHIE

Dr. Michael Greger *is a professional speaker on public health issues, particularly the benefits of a whole-food, plant-based diet, and the author of the international bestseller* How Not to Die.

Makes 1 serving

"Wake up your taste buds with this nutrient-dense smoothie featuring purple sweet potato, blackstrap molasses, peanut butter, and cocoa powder. For convenience, prebake several sweet potatoes so you have them on hand."

1 purple sweet potato, steamed until soft, then cooled	½ teaspoon ground cinnamon
	1 cup unsweetened soy milk
1 tablespoon peanut butter	1 cup frozen berries
1 tablespoon cocoa powder	1 tablespoon ground flaxseeds
1 tablespoon blackstrap molasses	

Combine all the ingredients in a high-speed blender and blend until smooth. Serve in a tall glass.

LEMON-INFUSED QUINOA BREAKFAST BOWL

Rip Esselstyn, *a former firefighter and triathlete, is an American health activist and author of such best-selling books as* The Engine 2 Diet, Plant-Strong, *and* The Engine 2 Seven-Day Rescue Diet.

Makes 2 servings

"Quinoa is the star of this breakfast bowl topped with a beautiful array of fresh fruit. You can vary the fruit according to what is available and what you have on hand."

½ cup quinoa	½ cup diced mango
½ cup unsweetened nondairy milk	½ cup raspberries
	½ cup chopped pineapple
1 teaspoon vanilla extract	2 cups baby spinach, chopped
1 lemon, zested	

Rinse quinoa thoroughly in a fine mesh strainer. Combine ½ cup water and nondairy milk in a medium saucepan and bring to a boil. Add the quinoa, vanilla extract, and half of the lemon zest. Stir, reduce the heat to low, cover, and simmer for about 15 minutes, or until the grain is translucent and the germ has spiraled out of each grain. Allow the quinoa to cool, then transfer to a large bowl. Add the mango, raspberries, pineapple, and remaining lemon zest. Toss to combine. Refrigerate for 30 minutes. Serve over the chopped baby spinach.

OVERNIGHT CHIA OATS WITH BERRIES

Michelle McMacken, M.D., *is a board-certified internal medicine physician who practices primary care in New York City, where she also teaches doctors in training and leads a plant-based lifestyle medicine program.*

Makes 1 serving

"This delicious and healthful breakfast can be quickly assembled the night before and ready to eat the next morning at home, or you can take it to work."

½ cup rolled oats

1 tablespoon chia seeds

¾ cup unsweetened nondairy milk, such as almond or soy milk

1 teaspoon vanilla extract

1 small banana, chopped

¼ cup walnuts (optional)

½ cup frozen berries

Combine the oats and chia seeds in a Mason jar (or other container with a tight-fitting lid) and shake to mix. Add the nondairy milk, vanilla extract, chopped banana, and walnuts, if using. Top with the frozen berries. Place the lid on the jar and refrigerate overnight. In the morning, it will be ready to enjoy.

POWERHOUSE OATS

Dr. Caldwell Esselstyn, Jr., *a former Olympic rowing gold medalist, directs the cardiovascular prevention and reversal program at the Cleveland Clinic Wellness Institute and is the author of the bestseller* Prevent and Reverse Heart Disease.

Makes 1 serving

"Oats reduce cholesterol, lower inflammation, and keep your blood sugar level in check. They should be part of everyone's breakfast. Any amount of oats and fruit can be used in this recipe, according to your preference and appetite. Avoid coconut milk or rice milk, or any milk with added oil."

¾ cup old-fashioned rolled oats, raw or cooked

1 cup mixed berries

1 small banana, sliced (optional)

1 tablespoon ground flax or chia seeds

¾ cup nondairy milk, such as almond, oat, or soy milk

Combine the oats and mixed berries in a bowl. Top with the banana, if using, and add flax or chia seeds. Pour in the nondairy milk to cover the oats and serve.

CHICKPEA OMELET

Charity Morgan *provides vegan meal preparation to several NFL players and has recently been featured on ESPN, highlighting her homemade meals that have encouraged athletes to improve their performance and overall health. Learn more at chefcharitymorgan.com.*

Makes 2 servings

"This has been my very favorite egg alternative. It's gluten free, soy free and has a great crepe-like texture. You can be creative and fill it with anything you would fill an egg omelet with. Note: Kala namak is a sulfurous salt that smells like egg! If you prefer not to use it, feel free to substitute the kala namak with pink Himalayan salt."

1 cup chickpea flour

1 cup unsweetened almond milk (or other nondairy milk)

1 tablespoon nutritional yeast

1 teaspoon kala namak or pink Himalayan salt

Cooking spray or 1 teaspoon avocado oil

Optional fillings: vegan cheese, sautéed mushrooms, vegan bacon or sausage, cooked spinach or kale, seitan, tofu, vegan chorizo, cooked potatoes, peppers, or onions

In a mixing bowl, combine the chickpea flour, almond milk, ¼ cup water, nutritional yeast, and kala namak. Whisk until smooth.

Spray a nonstick or cast-iron pan with cooking spray or avocado oil and heat over medium-high heat. Pour enough of the batter into the pan that it covers the bottom completely and forms a layer about ¼-inch thick. (If your pan is small or if you want to make two smaller omelets, divide the batter in half.) If you have a lot of excess liquid on top, pull one side of the omelet slightly back and allow the liquid to spill into the area you just pulled back (just as you would a traditional omelet). Reduce the heat to low and cover with a lid for 2 minutes. Remove the lid and top the omelet with the desired fillings. Fold one side over, turn off the heat, and place the lid back on to help ensure the vegan cheese is melted, if using. Serve.

Note: If you prefer a scramble instead of an omelet, follow each step, and instead of covering with a lid the first time, scramble just as you would eggs. You'll still want to cover the pan toward the end to make sure cheese melts, if using, and the flour is cooked through.

AIRPORT OATMEAL

> *An iconic musician, fierce animal rights activist, and owner of the plant-based Little Pine Restaurant in Silver Lake, Los Angeles,* **Moby** *is on a mission to save humanity via veganism.*

Makes 1 serving

"I've been a vegan for 31 years, and one of the biggest challenges as a vegan has always been eating well in airports. There's a Real Food Daily in Terminal 6 at LAX, but apart from that, it's almost impossible to find good vegan food, even in cosmopolitan international airports. So, based on years of being hungry in airports, I give you this profoundly simple, lifesaving, and intentionally vague recipe for airport oatmeal. Added bonus: None of these ingredients are problematic for TSA, so the hardworking men and women of the TSA won't be confiscating your food. It sounds almost painfully simple, but a healthy bowl of hot oatmeal with walnuts, raisins, and blueberries can be like a perfect, warm hug when you're waiting for a long flight."

½ cup quick oats	2 tablespoons walnuts
2 tablespoons raisins	2 tablespoons blueberries

Fill a plastic container with the oats, raisins, walnuts, and blueberries.

Then, as a modern day hunter-gatherer, wander the airport in search of hot water. Boiling water usually used for tea is the best, but in a pinch you can even use very hot water from a bathroom faucet. Add 1 cup of hot water to the oats and other ingredients. Stir well and enjoy.

APPETIZERS AND SNACKS

SPICY THAI MEATBALLS WITH ORANGE-CHILI DIPPING SAUCE

Del Sroufe *is a plant-based cooking instructor, public speaker and the author of four cookbooks including* Forks Over Knives: The Cookbook, *which remained on the* New York Times *best-seller list for 36 weeks.*

Makes 8 to 10 servings

"This recipe is one of my favorite party appetizers. It is easy to make, full of flavor, and has peanuts in it. How can you lose?! Note: You can also serve this over rice as a main dish for four."

¾ cup millet

1 small yellow onion, finely diced

4 cloves garlic, minced

1 tablespoon minced ginger

1 serrano pepper, minced

1 teaspoon sea salt

¼ teaspoon cayenne pepper (optional)

2 tablespoons peanut butter

¼ cup toasted peanuts, coarsely ground

½ cup orange juice

½ cup chili sauce

¼ cup brown rice syrup

2 tablespoons tamari

2 tablespoons rice vinegar

Zest of 1 orange

Combine 1½ cups water and millet in a small saucepan with a tight-fitting lid. Bring the mixture to a boil over high heat. Reduce the heat to medium-low and cook the millet for 20 minutes until it is very tender. If it is not tender, add another 2 to 3 tablespoons of water and let it cook another 5 minutes.

While the millet cooks, cook the onion in a large skillet over medium heat for 8 minutes, or until the onion starts to brown and turn translucent. Add the garlic, ginger, and serrano pepper, and cook for another minute.

Preheat the oven to 375 degrees Fahrenheit.

Add the cooked millet, salt, cayenne, peanut butter and ground peanuts to the pan and mix well.

Line a baking sheet with parchment paper. Using a small ice cream scoop or a tablespoon, shape the millet mixture into little balls and arrange them on the baking sheet. Bake for 20 minutes, or until the meatballs are firm to the touch and start to brown.

To make the orange-chili dipping sauce, combine the orange juice, chili sauce, brown rice syrup, tamari, rice vinegar, and orange zest in a small saucepan and bring to a boil over medium-low heat, stirring frequently. Remove from the heat and serve with the meatballs.

SWEET POTATO CORNBREAD

A graduate of North Carolina A&T State University, **Zakiyaa Michèl** is an Urban and Community Horticulture graduate, a self-taught chef, and a mad vegan-food scientist with a passion for food and plant-based advocacy.

Makes 9 to 12 servings

"This healthy take on classic cornbread features unexpected ingredients such as sweet potato, carrot juice, and apple butter."

- 3 medium sweet potatoes
- 5 tablespoons carrot juice
- 2 tablespoons ground flaxseed
- 1¼ cups coconut milk
- 2 tablespoons apple butter
- 1 tablespoon applesauce
- 1 cup all-purpose flour
- 1¼ cups yellow cornmeal
- 1 tablespoon baking powder
- ½ cup light brown sugar, lightly packed
- 1 teaspoon salt
- ½ teaspoon ground cinnamon
- ½ teaspoon ground nutmeg

Preheat the oven to 425 degrees Fahrenheit. Wash the sweet potatoes to remove any dirt, and poke each potato 3 to 4 times with a fork or knife on opposite sides. Do not peel. Microwave the sweet potatoes on high for 5 minutes. Flip each sweet potato over and microwave for another 5 minutes, or until wrinkly and slightly soft when squeezed with tongs. Set aside to cool.

Prepare a baking sheet by lining it with foil and setting a wire rack on top of the sheet. Place the microwaved sweet potatoes on the rack and roast until browned and very soft when squeezed with tongs, about 1 hour. Note that the sugar in the sweet potatoes will caramelize and may ooze out onto the sheet as they bake. Set aside for at least 10 minutes, or until the potatoes are cool enough to handle.

While the sweet potatoes are roasting, combine the carrot juice and ground flaxseed in a small bowl. Let sit at room temperature.

When the sweet potatoes are cool, peel away the potato skins by cutting a slit into the potato lengthwise and pushing the flesh into a small bowl. Repeat this process until all the sweet potato flesh is separated from the peel. Discard the peelings.

Puree the sweet potato flesh in a high-speed blender or food processor until smooth. Measure out 1 cup of the sweet potato puree and set aside. Store any remaining sweet potato puree for another use.

In a medium bowl, combine roasted sweet potato puree, coconut milk, apple butter, applesauce, and reserved carrot-flax mixture. Mix thoroughly.

In a large bowl, lightly sift the flour, cornmeal, baking powder, brown sugar, salt, cinnamon, and nutmeg. Mix thoroughly until combined.

Add the wet ingredients to the dry ingredients and stir until just combined, being careful not to overmix. Transfer the batter to a lightly oiled nonstick 9 x 9-inch pan or spoon it evenly into a lightly oiled muffin tin. Bake for 25 to 30 minutes, or until the cornbread is golden. Serve hot.

SRIRACHA–ALMOND BUTTER HUMMUS

Robin Robertson, *who has worked with food for more than 30 years as a restaurant chef and cooking teacher, is the author of more than 25 cookbooks, including* Vegan Planet, 1,000 Vegan Recipes, One-Dish Vegan, *and* Fresh from the Vegan Slow Cooker.

Makes about 2 cups

"Almond butter stands in for the traditional sesame paste in this flavorful, protein-rich dip that is enlivened by a jolt of sriracha. For a kid-friendly version, you can omit the sriracha and swap in peanut butter for the almond butter. Serve with cut veggies or whole-grain crackers."

One 15-ounce can chickpeas, drained and rinsed

1 large clove garlic, chopped

¼ cup almond butter

2 tablespoons fresh lemon juice

1 to 2 teaspoons sriracha sauce, to taste

½ teaspoon salt

1 tablespoon minced parsley or cilantro

Puree the chickpeas and garlic in a food processor until smooth. Add the almond butter, lemon juice, sriracha, and salt. Process until smooth and well blended. Add water, 1 teaspoon at a time, if a thinner consistency is desired.

Transfer the hummus to a small bowl and cover tightly. Refrigerate for at least an hour before serving to allow flavors to develop. Serve chilled or at room temperature topped with a sprinkling of parsley.

STUFFED GRAPE LEAVES

Marco Borges *is an exercise physiologist, the founder of* 22 Days Nutrition, *a* New York Times *best-selling author, and a plant-based living advocate. He is the author of* The Greenprint, The 22-Day Revolution, *and* The 22-Day Revolution Cookbook.

Makes 6 to 8 servings

"Making stuffed grape leaves is very time consuming but so worth it! These are uniquely made with quinoa, not with the traditional rice that is typically used, and this recipe has no oil. It's optional, so feel free to add ¼ cup of olive oil to the mixture if you desire, as well as a light drizzle after each layer. A full jar of grape leaves contains about 50 grape leaves, although some of the leaves may have broken in the jar or are too small to stuff. In any case, you will have enough to serve at least 6 to 8 people as part of a meal, or more if this is served as a party appetizer."

1 large yellow onion, peeled and cut crosswise into thirds

3 cups cooked quinoa

One 15-ounce can chickpeas, drained and rinsed

4 cloves garlic, minced

Juice of 2 lemons

1 cup minced fresh parsley

1 teaspoon dried mint leaves

½ teaspoon salt

One 16-ounce jar grape leaves

Dice one-third of the onion and transfer it to a food processor. Add the cooked quinoa, chickpeas, garlic, lemon, parsley, mint, and salt. Process to mix well. Set aside.

Slice the remaining two-thirds of the onion into large rings and arrange them on the bottom of a large pot. This will help prevent the grape leaves from potentially sticking to the pot.

Transfer the grape leaves to a mixing bowl. Gently open the leaves to prepare them for stuffing.

Add about a tablespoon of the quinoa mixture onto to each leaf and begin to wrap them up by folding in the sides of the leaf and gently rolling it up, being careful to prevent ripping.

Transfer the stuffed leaf to the pot on top of the onion rings. Repeat the steps using the remaining stuffing and leaves, arranging the stuffed leaves on the onion rings to create a consistent pattern when stacking. The first layer should be laid out in the same direction. The second layer should be in the opposite direction and so on. Sprinkle each layer with a pinch of salt and extra lemon juice. Repeat the steps until all the grape leaves are stuffed and stacked tightly in the pot.

Place a round plate on the top layer and press down, making sure the leaves are stacked tightly in the pot to prevent them from moving around and loosening when cooking. Add water in the pot until the water is about an inch or two above the plate. Add more weight on top of plate to make sure the leaves stay intact. Bring the water to a boil. Reduce the heat to medium-low and cook for about 30 minutes or until the water seems to have dried up. Remove from the heat and allow the grape leaves to steam for another 30 minutes. Serve.

BLACK BEAN–PUMPKIN QUESADILLAS WITH SWEET PEPPER SALSA AND LIME CREMA

A vegetable enthusiast and plant-based chef, **Andrea Nordby** *leads culinary development for Purple Carrot, the first 100 percent plant-based meal kit.*

Makes 6 to 8 servings

"These delicious quesadillas are as fun to make as they are to eat. In addition to serving as an appetizer for several people, they make a great lunch for two."

1 small onion, peeled and diced	3 tablespoons vegan sour cream
One 15-ounce can black beans, drained and rinsed	2 tablespoons chopped fresh cilantro
3 mini sweet peppers, seeded and diced	½ cup unsweetened pumpkin purée
1 lime, zested and halved	½ teaspoon ground cumin
Pinch of salt and pepper	Two 12-inch whole-wheat tortillas
1 jalapeño, trimmed, seeded, and minced	2 teaspoons cooking oil

To make the sweet pepper salsa, combine half of the diced onion, ¼ cup of the black beans, the diced peppers, juice from half the lime, and salt and pepper. Toss to combine. Set aside.

To make the lime crema, combine the lime zest, remaining lime juice, jalapeño, sour cream, cilantro, and a pinch of salt. Stir to blend. Set aside.

In a medium bowl, combine the remaining chopped onion, remaining black beans, pumpkin purée, cumin, and a pinch of salt and pepper.

Lay both tortillas flat on a work surface. Divide the black bean mixture between the tortillas and spread over one half. Fold the tortillas, pressing down to seal.

Heat 1 teaspoon of oil in a large skillet over medium-high heat. Once hot, add the first quesadilla. Cook until the bottom is golden brown, 2 to 3 minutes, then carefully flip to crisp the other side. Remove from the skillet and repeat with the remaining oil and the second quesadilla.

Cut each quesadilla into 4 pieces and transfer to a serving platter. Serve with the sweet pepper salsa and lime crema.

MAPLE-JERK HUMMUS

CC Péan *is an AfroCarib plant-based chef who utilizes African diaspora culinary heritage, foods, and cooking traditions to transform her clients' health.*

Makes 8 servings

"This is a spicy, sweet, Island spin on a Mediterranean staple. I like to season this hummus with Walkerswood Traditional Jamaican Jerk Seasoning Mild. For an interesting flavor combination, serve with jicama or sugar snap peas."

One 15-ounce can chickpeas, drained, liquid reserved

4 medium cloves garlic

⅓ cup good quality tahini

¾ teaspoon salt

4 tablespoons freshly squeezed lemon juice

½ tablespoon jerk seasoning, plus more for garnish

2 tablespoons maple syrup

¼ cup finely chopped sun-dried tomatoes in olive oil, oil reserved

¼ cup chopped scallions, divided

2 teaspoons olive oil

In a food processor, combine the drained chickpeas, garlic, tahini, salt, lemon juice, jerk seasoning, maple syrup, and ¼ cup of the chickpea liquid. Process for 5 minutes, stopping occasionally to scrape down the sides of the processor.

Add the sun-dried tomatoes and half of the scallions and process for 1 more minute, until you achieve the consistency you like. Transfer the hummus to a serving bowl. Garnish with a drizzle of olive oil and a sprinkle of dry jerk seasoning or a dollop of seasoning if using a paste, and the remaining scallions.

SOUPS

JACKFRUIT AND OKRA GUMBO

Darshana Thacker *is chef and culinary project manager for* Forks Over Knives. *A graduate of the Natural Gourmet Institute, she is the author of* Forks Over Knives: Flavor!

Makes 4 to 6 servings

"Gumbo is Southern comfort food that's packed with flavor. Many vegan versions have beans, but the jackfruit in this version gives it a nice hearty texture that absorbs the strong flavors from the spices. Shiitake mushrooms give it the umami flavor. Serve with corn bread or whole-wheat crackers."

½ cup all-purpose flour

Two 15-ounce cans water-packed jackfruit, drained, rinsed, and cut into ¾-inch pieces

2 tablespoons Creole spice mix

1½ teaspoons smoked paprika

2 medium onions, finely chopped

1 medium red bell pepper, finely chopped

2 stalks celery, finely chopped

1 cup shiitake mushroom, cut into long strips

1½ tablespoons minced garlic

2 teaspoons gumbo filé

1½ teaspoons dried thyme

½ teaspoon cayenne pepper

2 bay leaves

4 cups vegetable broth, divided

10 ounces frozen okra, thawed

1 cup cooked brown rice

½ cup minced fresh parsley leaves, plus more for garnish

Hot sauce (optional)

Pinch of sea salt

Pinch of ground black pepper

Roast the flour in a dry skillet over medium-low heat, stirring constantly for 5 minutes, until the flour turns light brown and gives out a toasty aroma. Set aside.

In a mixing bowl, combine the jackfruit, Creole spice mix, and paprika. Mix well to coat the jackfruit evenly with the seasoning. Set aside to marinate for 20 minutes.

In a large soup pot, combine the onions, bell pepper, celery, mushrooms, garlic, filé, thyme, cayenne, bay leaves, and ¼ cup of water. Cook over medium-low heat, stirring frequently, for 10 to 15 minutes, until the vegetables are tender. Add 1 to 2 tablespoons of the broth to keep the vegetables from sticking to the pot.

Remove the bay leaves from the pot and discard. In a bowl, mix the roasted flour with the remaining broth, using a whisk to blend and break up any clumps if formed.

Stir the broth mixture into the pot. Add the marinated jackfruit, okra, rice, and parsley. Cook for 10 to 15 minutes, until the flavors merge and the stew thickens.

Add the hot sauce, if using, and salt and black pepper to taste. Taste and adjust seasoning.

Garnish with parsley and serve warm.

BLOOMING BLACK BEAN SOUP

Queen Afua
Makes 6 to 8 servings

"It is important to soak beans in water overnight (or longer) to help prevent gas when beans are consumed. If the soaking water is poured off and refreshed more than once (over a day and a half), the beans will begin to sprout and will offer more nutrients and become easier to digest when eaten."

2 cups dried black beans

1 cup chopped celery

1 cup chopped raw okra

1 cup chopped scallions

2 teaspoons ground turmeric

2 teaspoons ground cumin

1 to 2 teaspoons sea salt or pink Himalayan salt

1 cup chopped basil (optional)

1 sprig fresh sage

Optional garnishes: chopped parsley or cilantro and minced scallions or chives

Soak the dried black beans overnight in a glass bowl with enough water to cover the beans. Drain the beans and transfer them to a large cast-iron or stainless-steel pot. Add 4 cups of water and bring to a boil, then reduce the heat to a low simmer, cover, and cook for 30 to 45 minutes. Check on the beans frequently so they don't burn. The beans are done when they are soft to fork touch and cooked all the way through. Remove the pot of cooked beans from the hot stove.

Stir the celery, okra, and scallions into the pot with the beans, then add the turmeric, cumin, salt, basil, if using, and the sage. Let the hot beans absorb the flavors of the fresh ingredients.

When ready to serve, spoon the soup into bowls and add garnishes, if using.

CREAMY TOMATO BASIL BISQUE

Del Sroufe

Makes 4 servings

"This creamy soup combines fresh and sun-dried tomatoes to add a depth of flavor. Be sure your nondairy milk is plain and unsweetened to use in this savory bisque."

1 large yellow onion, finely diced	½ cup fresh basil, minced
2 stalks celery, finely diced	2 cups diced tomatoes
2 carrots, peeled and finely diced	¼ cup chopped sun-dried tomatoes
4 cloves minced garlic	2 cups unsweetened nondairy milk
1 teaspoon dried thyme leaves	2 tablespoons arrowroot powder

Combine the onion, celery, and carrots in a large saucepan over medium heat. Sauté for 7 to 8 minutes, adding water, 1 to 2 tablespoons at a time, to keep the vegetables from sticking to the pan. Add the garlic, thyme, basil, tomatoes, and sun-dried tomatoes. Cover and cook for 15 minutes, stirring occasionally.

In a small bowl, whisk together the nondairy milk and arrowroot until blended. Add the arrowroot mixture to the pot and stir to mix well. Remove the saucepan from the heat. Working in batches, carefully transfer the soup to a high-speed blender with a tight-fitting lid covered with a towel and purée until the soup is blended. Return the puréed soup to the pan and heat if needed.

BAD ASS VEGAN SWEET POTATO SOUP

John Lewis's *love for his community brought forth the brainchild VeganSmart, a plant-based protein shake company with a foundation whose mission is to prevent obesity through education, physical activity, and plant-based nutrition.*

Makes 4 servings

"I created this soup for those that are stuck in the cold weather. I made the raw version, which warmed up well in my Vitamix blender, but for those who want the cooked version, feel free to put this on the stovetop and heat up to your liking."

1 large sweet potato, peeled and chopped

1 large carrot, sliced

3 dates, pitted

½ ripe Hass avocado, peeled and pitted

2 cloves garlic

⅓ small jalapeño chili

⅓ onion, chopped

In a high-speed blender, combine the sweet potato, carrot, dates, avocado, garlic, chili, and 2 cups water. Blend on low and then gradually increase the power as the ingredients begin to combine, for 2 to 5 minutes, until very smooth.

Transfer to bowls to serve, garnished with the onion (see Note). If you prefer to cook the soup, transfer the soup to a saucepan and simmer until hot.

Note: If you prefer not to use the onion as garnish, you can blend it with the other ingredients in the blender.

CREAM OF ZUCCHINI-KALE SOUP

Nina Curtis, *the director and executive chef for the Adventist Health, Roseville Campus Café and Culinary Arts department, is a leader and trailblazer in the plant-based culinary movement.*

Makes 4 servings

"No cooking needed to make this refreshing soup. Simply combine all the ingredients in a high-speed blender, and it's ready to go. Store the soup in a sealed container in the refrigerator, where it will keep for up to three days."

2 medium zucchinis, peeled and chopped

2 celery ribs, chopped

2 to 3 cups chopped kale leaves, packed

2 small cloves garlic, crushed

2 tablespoons lemon juice

2 tablespoons extra-virgin olive oil

2 teaspoons white miso

½ teaspoon sea salt, or to taste

Pinch of cayenne

1 ripe avocado, peeled, pitted, and mashed

2 tablespoons minced fresh dill

Combine 1 cup water, zucchini, celery, kale, garlic, lemon juice, olive oil, miso, salt, and cayenne in a high-speed blender and process until smooth. Add the avocado and dill and blend briefly. If a thinner soup is desired, blend in additional water, 1 teaspoon at a time, to achieve the desired consistency. Serve chilled, at room temperature, or slightly warm.

PEPPER-POT SOUP

Raymond Jackson, *an accomplished chef with extensive international experience, is currently working in Memphis, Tennessee, as executive chef at Crosstown Arts Cafe, a plant-based restaurant.*

Makes 8 to 10 servings

"The long culinary heritage of pepper-pot soup began in West Africa before making its way to the West Indies and the Caribbean, and on up to Atlantic coast cities of North America. Today, various versions of pepper-pot soup remain popular in Jamaica and other areas of the Caribbean, as well as in Charleston, South Carolina, and Philadelphia."

1 medium butternut squash	1½ quarts vegetable broth
¼ cup vegan butter	1 large sweet potato, peeled and diced
2 tablespoons brown sugar	
1½ teaspoons ground cinnamon	Two 13.5-ounce cans unsweetened coconut milk
1 teaspoon ground allspice	
4 cloves	1 or 2 Scotch bonnet chilies, to taste
1 tablespoon olive oil	
1 red bell pepper, diced	2 sprigs fresh thyme
1 green bell pepper, diced	2 bay leaves
1 medium yellow onion, diced	8 ounces baby spinach
Salt and ground black pepper, to taste	Pinch of Jamaican pepper sauce (optional)

Preheat the oven to 350 degrees Fahrenheit. Cut the squash in half and remove and discard the seeds. Rub the cut side of the squash with the butter, brown sugar, cinnamon, allspice, and cloves. Arrange the squash halves in a large baking dish, cut side up, and cover tightly with aluminum foil. Roast until very soft, about 90 minutes. Set aside to cool.

Heat the oil in a large soup pot over medium heat. Add the bell peppers and onion and season with salt and pepper to taste. Cook for 5 minutes to soften. Add the vegetable broth and sweet potato and bring to a boil. Reduce the heat to a low simmer and add 1 can of the coconut milk and the Scotch bonnet chilies, thyme, and bay leaves. Simmer gently until the vegetables are tender, about 20 minutes. (Do not boil or the chilies may burst and the soup may be too spicy.)

While the soup is simmering, scrape the cooled roasted butternut squash pulp from the skin, discarding the cloves and skin. Transfer the squash pulp to a high-speed blender and puree with the second can of coconut milk until smooth. Add the squash purée and the spinach to the soup and cook for a few minutes until the spinach is wilted. When ready to serve, remove and discard the Scotch bonnet, thyme sprigs, and bay leaves. Taste the soup and adjust the seasonings with salt, pepper, and Jamaican pepper sauce, if desired.

VEGETABLE SOUP

Mother of six children, **Dorothy Adams,** *who has spent 30 years in the food industry as the head cook for Amstead Day Care Center, changed her diet after years of suffering from diabetes and other health-related issues.*

Makes 8 servings

"You can change up the vegetables in this basic soup according to your preference and what's on hand. For a richer flavor, blend a spoonful of vegan bouillon paste into a cup of hot water and add to the soup before salting the broth."

1 tablespoon olive oil

2 large red onions, chopped

1 cup chopped celery

1 cup chopped carrots

1 large sweet potato, diced

2 green bell peppers, diced

2 red bell peppers, diced

10 cloves garlic, minced

Salt and ground black pepper, to taste

2 large basil leaves

2 medium bay leaves

1 cup whole-grain elbow macaroni

2 cups fresh spinach

Heat the oil in a large soup pot over medium heat. Add the onions, celery, carrots, sweet potato, bell peppers, and garlic. Season with salt and pepper and cook, stirring until the vegetables are softened, about 10 minutes. Add the basil leaves and bay leaves, stir in enough water to cover, and bring to a boil. Reduce the heat to a simmer and cook until the vegetables are tender. Taste and adjust the seasoning, adding more salt, if needed. Add the macaroni to the soup and continue cooking until tender, about 10 minutes. Just before serving, stir in the spinach. Serve hot.

THAI SWEET POTATO SOUP

Chef Ayinde, *a lifelong vegan and 21-year veteran vegan chef, lives in Los Angeles, where he sells his flagship product (Mac & Yease) at 63 stores and nationwide online via ieatgrass.com.*

Makes 4 servings

"This rich and creamy soup has a nice touch of heat thanks to the serrano chili. If you prefer a milder soup, use only half of the chili or leave it out."

2 tablespoons cooking oil

½ cup diced yellow onion

½ cup diced celery

2 tablespoons grated fresh garlic

2 tablespoons chopped fresh ginger

2 cups diced sweet potatoes

1 serrano chili, seeded and chopped (optional)

2 tablespoons coconut cream

Sea salt, to taste

Heat the oil in a soup pot over medium-high heat. Add the onions, celery, garlic, and ginger and cook, stirring until the onions become translucent, 3 to 5 minutes. Add the sweet potatoes, chili, if using, and 3 cups of water and bring to a boil. Reduce the heat to a simmer and cook until the sweet potatoes become fork tender, about 30 minutes.

Transfer the soup mixture to a high-speed blender. Add the coconut cream and blend until smooth. Return the soup back into the pot. Season with salt to taste. Serve hot.

SALADS

CAMERON CAESAR SALAD WITH SUZY'S CAESAR DRESSING

An environmental advocate, mom of five, and author of OMD: The Simple, Plant-Based Program to Save Your Health and Save the Planet, **Suzy Amis Cameron** *is focused on plant-based food solutions to address climate change and improve health.*

Makes 4 servings

"The key to a great Caesar salad is a great dressing. Unfortunately, a traditional Caesar dressing is loaded with anchovies and raw eggs. No need to worry; you can indulge deliciously with my (amazing) Caesar dressing."

3 cloves garlic

1 tablespoon capers, drained

1 cup vegan mayonnaise

1 tablespoon white miso paste

2 tablespoons nutritional yeast flakes

½ tablespoon light agave nectar

2 tablespoons fresh lemon juice

1 cup olive oil

Salt and ground black pepper, to taste

3 cups day-old bread, cubed

3 tablespoons olive oil

1 teaspoon garlic powder

½ teaspoon salt

¼ teaspoon ground black pepper

1 large head romaine lettuce, well washed and dried

To make the Caesar dressing, combine the garlic, capers, mayonnaise, miso paste, nutritional yeast, agave nectar, lemon juice, and ¼ cup water in a food processor. Pulse to blend. With the motor still running, slowly add the oil in a thin stream. Add salt and pepper to taste. Blend until smooth. Set aside.

Preheat the oven to 375 degrees Fahrenheit. To make the croutons, toss the bread cubes with olive oil, garlic powder, salt, and pepper. Arrange the seasoned bread cubes in a single layer on a baking sheet. Bake, tossing occasionally, until the croutons are golden, 12 to 15 minutes.

While the croutons are baking, tear the lettuce into bite-size pieces and place in a large salad bowl. Toss with the croutons and the dressing and serve.

SUPER GREEN LIVE SALAD AND AVOCADO DRESSING

Queen Afua

Makes 3 to 4 servings

"Enjoy this live salad as a side dish or a main dish. If you don't own a spiralizer, zucchini noodles can be purchased premade from the supermarket. If you like, you can add some cayenne or paprika to the Cajun seasoning. Whenever possible, use fresh herbs instead of the dried version. The avocado dressing can also be used as a dip with organic corn chips or spread on organic crackers."

1 cup finely chopped arugula

1 cup finely chopped callaloo or spinach

1 cup finely chopped kale

1 cup chopped leeks

1 cup chopped basil

1 cup chopped watercress

1 cup zucchini noodles

1 or 2 medium-sized, well-ripened avocados, rinsed

1 cup sun-dried tomatoes

½ cup cold-pressed olive oil

2 teaspoons Cajun seasoning, or to taste

1 to 2 teaspoons sea salt or pink Himalayan salt

Juice of 1 lime

Sprig of thyme

Layer the arugula, callaloo, kale, leeks, basil, watercress, and zucchini noodles in a large bowl. Cover the bowl with a kitchen towel and set aside.

To make the avocado dressing, pit and peel the avocados, then scoop out the pulp and transfer to a high-speed blender or food processor. Add the sun-dried tomatoes, olive oil, Cajun seasoning, sea salt, lime juice, and thyme. Blend until smooth and creamy. Pour as much dressing as desired onto the salad greens. Use your fingers to massage the dressing into the greens. Transfer any leftover dressing into a glass bottle or jar and store in the refrigerator.

ROASTED BEET AND POTATO SALAD

Jenné Claiborne, *a vegan chef, blogger, and author of the* Sweet Potato Soul *cookbook, is known for creating healthy and easy-to-make vegan recipes, and for veganizing soul-food classics.*

Makes 2 to 3 servings

"You can double the lemon vinaigrette recipe to make plenty of dressing to last the week."

Juice of 2 lemons

1 tablespoon Dijon mustard

2 teaspoons maple syrup

1 teaspoon minced garlic

1½ teaspoons sea salt

¼ cup extra-virgin olive oil

2 medium Yukon gold potatoes, diced

2 large beets, peeled and diced

1 tablespoon grapeseed oil

1 teaspoon minced fresh oregano

½ teaspoon ground black pepper

2 to 3 small heads lettuce, chopped

One 15-ounce can white beans, drained and rinsed

¼ cup toasted pepitas

To make the dressing, combine the lemon juice, Dijon mustard, maple syrup, garlic, ½ teaspoon sea salt, and olive oil in a small bowl and stir to combine. Set aside.

Preheat the oven to 375 degrees Fahrenheit. Line a baking sheet with a silicone baking mat or parchment paper.

Toss the cubed potatoes and beets with the grapeseed oil, then spread them evenly onto the baking sheet. Sprinkle with oregano, 1 teaspoon sea salt, and pepper. Roast for 35 minutes.

Place the lettuce into a large mixing bowl. Add the roasted vegetables and beans. Top with about half of the dressing and toss well. Top with more dressing and season with salt. Garnish with pepitas before serving.

EAT WHAT ELEPHANTS EAT BOWL

Dominick Thompson *is a leader in the vegan community and founder of Crazies and Weirdos, a successful New York–based startup that produces hip, sustainable clothing made in New York from recycled and organic materials.*

Makes 2 servings

"Next level plant-based eating is here to enjoy with this iconic signature bowl from Eat What Elephants Eat. Be sure to rinse and scrub your vegetables well before making this recipe."

¼ teaspoon chili powder

1¼ teaspoons garlic powder

½ teaspoon onion powder

¼ teaspoon paprika

1 Japanese sweet potato

1 bunch kale

1½ cups cooked or canned chickpeas, drained

2 tablespoons liquid aminos or soy sauce, divided

1 tablespoon fresh lemon juice, divided

Salt and ground black pepper, to taste

1 cup chopped tempeh

1 large ripe tomato, diced

1 avocado, peeled, pitted, and halved

1 cup shelled pistachios

2 tablespoons hemp seeds

1 tablespoon black cumin seeds (nigella seeds) (optional)

½ cup vegan mayonnaise

2 tablespoons apple cider vinegar

1½ teaspoons dried dill

1 teaspoon dried parsley

¼ teaspoon paprika

¼ teaspoon sea salt

¾ teaspoon maple syrup

In a small bowl, combine the chili powder, ¼ teaspoon garlic powder, ¼ teaspoon onion powder, and paprika. Set aside.

Preheat the oven to 400 degrees Fahrenheit. Poke holes in the sweet potato 3 to 4 times with a fork, and bake for 50 to 60 minutes, until soft. Remove the sweet potato from the oven and let it sit for 2 minutes to cool slightly. While still warm, cut the potato into slices or bite-sized pieces.

Strip the kale from stems and divide the kale equally into two bowls. Distribute the sliced sweet potato equally between the two bowls of kale.

Heat a medium skillet over medium heat. Add the chickpeas and 1 tablespoon of the liquid aminos, then season with ½ teaspoon of the reserved seasoning mix, ½ tablespoon lemon juice, and salt and pepper to taste. Sauté for 7 to 10 minutes until the chickpeas begin to become firmer. Distribute the chickpeas equally between the bowls of kale.

Reheat the same skillet over medium heat. Add the tempeh, 3 tablespoons of water, the remaining 1 tablespoon of liquid aminos, and the remaining ½ tablespoon of lemon juice. Season the tempeh with the remaining ½ teaspoon of the seasoning mix and salt and pepper to taste. Cook for 7 to 10 minutes, stirring to coat the tempeh with the spices.

Distribute the tempeh between the two salad bowls. Arrange one avocado half onto each bowl. Sprinkle the pistachio nuts, hemp seeds, and black cumin seeds, if using, evenly between both bowls.

Combine the vegan mayonnaise, apple cider vinegar, dill, 1 teaspoon garlic powder, parsley, ¼ teaspoon onion powder, paprika, ground black pepper, sea salt, and maple syrup in a separate bowl and whisk until well blended. Top each of the salad bowls with the dressing and serve.

TACO SALAD

Taymer Mason *is a vegan chef, the best-selling cookbook author of* Caribbean Vegan, *and a food scientist with a special interest in soy- and gluten-free plant proteins and clean personal-care products. Check out her website at www.islandlovegourmet.com.*

Makes 4 servings

"This is a healthier way to enjoy tacos. If you cannot use oats, you can substitute with cooked wild rice instead."

2 cups kale, tough stems removed

Juice of ½ lemon

1 tablespoon olive oil

2¼ teaspoons pink salt

1 medium head Romaine lettuce, chopped

1 jalapeño chili, thinly sliced

1 cup grape tomatoes, halved lengthwise

1 small ripe avocado, peeled, pitted, and diced

2 large portobello mushrooms caps, chopped

½ cup walnuts

1 large onion, chopped

1 teaspoon ground cumin

½ teaspoon chili powder

1 teaspoon garlic powder

5 tablespoons coconut oil

1½ cups old-fashioned rolled oats

1 clove garlic, crushed

1 tablespoon chopped fresh cilantro

¼ teaspoon ground black pepper

¼ teaspoon salt

Tear the kale into small pieces and place them into a large salad bowl. Add the lemon juice, olive oil, and ¼ teaspoon pink salt, and massage it with your hands until it is wilted. Add the lettuce, jalapeño, tomatoes, and avocado, and toss to combine. Set aside.

In a food processor, combine the mushrooms, walnuts, onion, 2 teaspoons pink salt, cumin, chili powder, and garlic powder. Pulse to combine and finely mince the mixture. Heat 2 tablespoons coconut oil in a large skillet over medium heat. Add the mushroom mixture and stir in the oats. Reduce the heat to low and cook for 20 minutes, stirring frequently, until the mixture is cooked. Taste for salt and adjust the seasonings if needed. Set aside to cool before placing it on the salad.

In a small bowl, combine the garlic, cilantro, 3 tablespoons of coconut oil, black pepper, and salt. Drizzle the dressing over the salad and serve immediately.

MAIN DISHES

OVEN-ROASTED MOROCCAN SQUASH WITH TAHINI SAUCE

CC Péan

Makes 2 to 4 servings

"This flavorful squash is like a delicious, comforting trip to North Africa. Serve over your favorite grain for a main dish meal or alone as a side dish. Ras el hanout is a spice blend that features coriander, cinnamon, cumin, allspice, ginger, turmeric, and black pepper. Look for it online or in well-stocked markets."

1 medium-size Kabocha squash, peeled, seeded, and cut into 2-inch pieces

3 tablespoons extra-virgin olive oil

2 teaspoons ras el hanout spice

½ teaspoon salt, plus more for seasoning

⅓ cup tahini

2 tablespoons fresh lemon juice

½ teaspoon finely minced garlic

4 cups cooked brown rice

½ bunch parsley, leaves only, coarsely chopped

Preheat the oven to 400 degrees Fahrenheit. Line a baking sheet with parchment paper and set aside.

Place the squash pieces in a large bowl and drizzle it with 2 tablespoons olive oil. Add the spice and salt and toss until evenly distributed.

Spread the squash on the baking sheet in a single layer, taking care not to crowd the pieces together. If necessary, use two baking sheets. Bake for 30 minutes.

In a bowl combine the tahini, lemon juice, 1 tablespoon of olive oil, and garlic. Whisk the ingredients together until they start to combine. Drizzle up to ¼ cup water to thin the mixture. When it reaches the consistency of salad dressing, it's ready. Taste and add more salt if needed. Whisk again to incorporate. Set aside.

Spoon the roasted squash onto a bed of hot cooked rice. Drizzle with the tahini sauce and sprinkle with the chopped parsley.

HOPPIN' JOHN STEW

Darshana Thacker

Makes 6 servings

"Black-eyed peas are not a frequently used legume, but they take center stage in this version of the classic Hoppin' John stew. This stew is so well flavored that you may view the black-eyed pea in a whole new way. If you can't find liquid smoke, you can substitute 1 teaspoon smoked paprika."

1 medium onion, cut into ¼-inch dice

2 cups trumpet mushrooms, cut into ½-inch dice

4 stalks celery, cut into ¼-inch dice

1 red bell pepper, cut into ¼-inch dice

1½ tablespoons minced garlic

1½ tablespoons Cajun seasoning

3 cups vegetable broth, divided

One 28-ounce can fire-roasted tomatoes

1 bunch collard greens or kale, chopped

2 to 3 bay leaves

1½ teaspoons dried thyme

¼ teaspoon liquid smoke

Three 15-ounce cans black-eyed peas, drained and rinsed

2 tablespoons white wine vinegar

Pinch of sea salt

Pinch of ground black pepper

2 tablespoons finely chopped scallions

6 cups cooked brown rice

Heat a large saucepan over high heat. Add the onion, mushrooms, celery, peppers, garlic, and Cajun seasoning, and cook for 10 minutes, stirring frequently. Add ¼ cup of the vegetable broth, as needed, to prevent the vegetables from sticking.

Stir in the tomatoes, greens, bay leaves, thyme, liquid smoke, and the remaining broth. Bring to a boil and cook for 15 minutes, or until the greens are tender. Remove the bay leaves.

Add the black-eyed peas, vinegar, and salt and pepper to taste. Cover and simmer for 10 minutes until the stew thickens.

Garnish with scallions and serve warm with brown rice.

SWEET POTATO ENCHILADAS WITH CASHEW-CHILI SOUR CREAM

The mission of brothers **Chad and Derek Sarno** *(founders of Wicked Healthy Food) is to drive plant-based culinary innovation on a global level and to empower people with accessible and delicious food that's free from animals.*

Makes 6 servings

"Don't let the long list of ingredients deter you from making these fabulous enchiladas. Make the components ahead of time and they can be assembled quickly."

1 cup raw cashews

2 tablespoons fresh lime juice

2 tablespoons nutritional yeast

3 jalapeño chilies, halved lengthwise, seeded, stems and top removed, plus more for garnish

¾ cup fresh cilantro leaves, plus more for garnish

1 teaspoon sea salt, divided

2 teaspoons ground black pepper

2 zucchinis, cut into half-moons ¼-inch thick

2 cups peeled and cubed sweet potatoes

2 red bell peppers, seeded and diced

1 yellow bell pepper, seeded and diced

2 onions, finely chopped

¼ cup sliced green onion

½ cup chopped fresh flat leaf parsley

1 tablespoon ground cumin

1 teaspoon garlic powder

2 teaspoons onion powder

½ cup low-sodium vegetable broth

Cooking spray, for baking sheet

One 28-ounce can tomatoes, pureed in high-speed blender until smooth

One 4-ounce can green hatch chilies, drained

¼ cup tomato paste

1 tablespoon minced fresh garlic

12 whole-grain flour tortillas

3 limes, cut into wedges, for squeezing

To make the cashew-chili sour cream, soak the raw cashews in enough warm water to cover them, for at least 3 hours or overnight. Rinse, drain, and transfer to a high-speed blender. Add the lime juice, nutritional yeast, jalapeño, ¼ cup cilantro, ½ teaspoon sea salt, and ½ teaspoon black pepper and blend until silky smooth, 4 to 5 minutes. As you blend, add up to ½ cup water until you have a creamy, pourable sauce. Use immediately or refrigerate for up to 3 days.

Preheat the oven to 375 degrees Fahrenheit. Toss the zucchini, sweet potato, 1 red bell pepper and the yellow bell pepper, 1 onion, parsley, 1 tablespoon cumin, 1 teaspoon black pepper, garlic powder, onion powder, ½ teaspoon sea salt, and vegetable broth in a large bowl until well coated.

Lightly oil a baking sheet and add the sweet potato mixture. Roast in the oven until browned and soft enough to cut with a fork, 35 to 45 minutes, stirring several times. Remove from the oven and cover to keep warm.

Chop and deseed 1 jalapeño. Combine the tomatoes, chilies, tomato paste, remaining onion, 1 red bell pepper, jalapeño, cumin, garlic, ½ cup cilantro, and remaining ½ teaspoon black pepper in a medium saucepan and heat on medium-low heat for 30 to 35 minutes, stirring frequently. Remove from heat and set aside.

Warm the tortillas directly in a hot pan. Spread about ½ cup sweet potato mixture filling through the center of each tortilla, then fold tortilla sides over the filling. Place two enchiladas on a plate, seam side down. Repeat with the remaining tortillas and filling. Smother the enchiladas with tomato sauce and cashew-chili sour cream.

Garnish with chopped chilies and cilantro. Serve with lime wedges for squeezing.

PASTA WITH KALE AND SAUSAGE

Huntsville, Alabama native **Donna Green-Goodman,** *a public health educator, is a plant-based diet advocate and the author of* Somethin' to Shout About!

Makes 6 to 8 servings

"This hearty meal comes together quickly. If you can't find the brand-name products listed, you can substitute with different brands of vegan sausage and nondairy products."

2 tablespoons olive oil

2 Beyond Meat Hot Italian Sausages, sliced

1 onion, sliced

½ red bell pepper, sliced

½ yellow bell pepper, sliced

½ orange bell pepper, sliced

2 cloves garlic, minced

2 to 3 cups chopped fresh kale

1 to 2 cups sliced mushrooms

1 teaspoon dried oregano

1 teaspoon dried basil

1 teaspoon Italian seasoning

Salt, to taste

16 ounces whole-grain or gluten-free spaghetti

½ to 1 cup Ripple Plant-Based Half & Half

1 teaspoon McKay's Chicken Style Instant Broth and Seasoning

4 ounces Daiya Mozzarella Style Shreds

Heat the oil in a large skillet over medium heat. Add the sausage slices and cook until browned, about 5 minutes, turning once halfway through. Add the onion, bell peppers, and garlic and sauté for 3 to 5 minutes, or until the onion is softened. Add kale and mushrooms and cook for 5 minutes, or until the vegetables are tender. Add the oregano, basil, Italian seasoning, and salt to taste, and toss to combine. Keep warm.

Cook the pasta in a pot of boiling salted water until it is just tender. Reserve 1 cup of the cooking water, then drain the pasta and return it to the pot. Add the nondairy half and half, the reserved pasta water, and the broth and seasoning, stirring to combine. Add the cooked vegetables, sausage, and mozzarella to the pasta and mix to combine. Taste and adjust the seasonings as needed. Serve hot.

POLENTA STACKS WITH BLACK BEAN AND CORN SALSA

Robin Robertson

Makes 3 servings

"Ready-to-use polenta is available in vacuum sealed tubes, making it easy to cut into thin slices. Made with on-hand ingredients, this dinner can be assembled in minutes but looks (and tastes) great."

One 18-ounce package precooked polenta

1 tablespoon olive oil

One 16-ounce jar mild tomato salsa

One 15.5-ounce can black beans, rinsed and drained

1 cup fresh or thawed frozen corn kernels

2 tablespoons pickled jalapeños, drained

1 teaspoon chili powder

½ teaspoon onion powder

Salt and ground black pepper, to taste

1 ripe avocado, peeled, pitted, and diced

Preheat the oven to 350 degrees Fahrenheit. Line a rimmed baking sheet with parchment paper or a silicone mat. Cut the polenta into slices about 1/2-inch thick (you should get 12 slices). Brush the polenta slices with the olive oil and arrange them on the prepared baking sheet. Bake for 10 minutes to heat through.

While the polenta is baking, combine the remaining ingredients except the avocado in a saucepan over medium heat. Cook, stirring, until the mixture is hot and well combined, about 5 minutes.

To serve, arrange two polenta slices on each plate. Spoon some of the black bean mixture over the polenta and top each with another slice of polenta. Top each stack with more of the black bean mixture, followed by another polenta slice, and the remaining black bean mixture. Top each stack with diced avocado and serve.

ROASTED VEGGIE LASAGNA

> **Dotsie Bausch**, *a powerful influencer for plant-based eating for athletes and nonathletes alike, is a seven-time USA Cycling National Champion, a two-time Pan American Champion, and an Olympic silver medalist in women's track cycling.*

Makes 6 to 8 servings

"Use fresh lasagna noodles, if you can find them. If you use dried lasagna noodles, you should partially boil them before assembling the lasagna."

1½ pounds zucchini, thinly sliced lengthwise

2 pounds button mushrooms, sliced

Two 16-ounce containers firm tofu, drained

Salt and ground black pepper, to taste

⅓ cup nutritional yeast

1 teaspoon chopped garlic

1½ tablespoons lemon juice

2 teaspoons dried oregano

1 tablespoon extra-virgin olive oil

3 cups vegan marinara sauce

16 ounces whole-wheat fresh lasagna noodles

½ cup fresh basil leaves

Preheat the oven to 400 degrees Fahrenheit. Line a rimmed baking pan with parchment paper or a silicone mat. Arrange the zucchini, mushrooms, and tofu in the pan and season with salt and pepper. Roast for 25 minutes, or until the vegetables are tender and just beginning to brown. Remove from the oven and reduce heat to 350 degrees Fahrenheit.

When the tofu is cool enough to handle, crumble the tofu finely into a large mixing bowl. Add the nutritional yeast, garlic, lemon juice, oregano, olive oil, salt, and black pepper.

Lightly oil a large lasagna pan. Spread ½ cup marinara sauce over the bottom of the pan. Arrange 4 fresh or cooked lasagna noodles over the sauce and top the noodles with half of the roasted vegetables. Spread half of the tofu mixture over the vegetables. Arrange 4 noodles and 1 cup of marinara sauce over the tofu. Cover the marinara sauce with the remaining roasted vegetables and tofu. Cover this layer with the 4 remaining lasagna noodles and the remaining marinara sauce. (The top should be red with marinara as the top layer.)

Cover the lasagna tightly with aluminum foil and bake for 30 minutes. Uncover and bake 15 minutes longer, or until the noodles are crisping at the edges and everything is bubbling gently. Remove from the oven and arrange the basil leaves over the top of the lasagna. Cut and serve.

CHIPOTLE MAC 'N' CHEESE

Megan Sadd *is a vegan chef, wellness leader, the author of* 30-Minute Vegan Dinners: 75 Fast Plant-Based Meals You're Going to Crave, *and star of her website and video channel,* Carrots & Flowers.

Makes 4 servings

"Soak the cashews for 4 hours or overnight to soften, then drain. You can also boil the cashews for 10 minutes if you're short on time."

2 cups brown rice pasta shells	2 tablespoons nutritional yeast
¼ cup soaked cashews	1 teaspoon smoked paprika
¼ cup hemp seeds	¾ teaspoon salt
¼ teaspoon ground chipotle powder	½ cup cooked vegan bacon, finely chopped (optional)
1 tablespoon tomato paste	⅓ cup gluten-free panko crumbs
½ teaspoon apple cider vinegar	½ cup vegan cheddar shreds (optional)
1 teaspoon agave nectar	
3 tablespoons tapioca flour	2 tablespoons finely chopped chives, to garnish

Preheat the oven to 425 degrees Fahrenheit. Cook the pasta in a pot of boiling salted water for 8 minutes, then drain and set aside.

Combine the soaked cashews, hemp seeds, chipotle powder, tomato paste, apple cider vinegar, agave nectar, tapioca flour, nutritional yeast, paprika, salt, and 1½ cups of water in a high-speed blender. Blend on high for 2 minutes until smooth and creamy.

Heat a saucepan over medium-high heat. Transfer the cashew mixture to the hot saucepan. Begin stirring right away, scraping the sides and bottom of the pot to prevent sticking. Stir for 2 to 3 minutes, or until the lumps are mostly gone, then add the cooked pasta to the saucepan. Add the vegan bacon, if using, and mix well to combine.

Transfer the pasta to a lightly oiled 8 x 8-inch baking dish. Top with the panko crumbs and vegan cheddar shreds, if using. Bake until the top is nicely browned, 8 to 10 minutes. Remove from the oven and sprinkle with the chives. Let cool for 3 to 5 minutes before serving.

QUINOA AND TEMPEH STIR-FRY WITH BROCCOLI AND CARROTS

Gregory Brown, *who wanted his restaurant to have its roots in a city of community, opened Baltimore's The Land of Kush in 2011. He currently sits on the board of the Visit Baltimore Foundation and the Black Vegetarian Society of Maryland.*

Makes 4 to 6 servings

"This simple but satisfying stir-fry hits all the right notes with its combination of sesame-soy seasoned tempeh, fluffy quinoa, and tender broccoli and carrots."

2 cups quinoa, well rinsed

2 tablespoons dark sesame oil

One 8-ounce pack of tempeh, cubed

3 cups chopped onion

2 tablespoons minced garlic

Salt and ground black pepper, to taste

3 cups chopped carrots

4 cups small broccoli florets

2 tablespoons soy sauce

Combine the quinoa and 4 cups of water in a saucepan and bring to a boil. Reduce the heat to a simmer and cook the quinoa until it is tender and the water is evaporated, about 20 minutes. (If any water remains, drain the quinoa.) Set aside.

Heat the sesame oil in a wok or large skillet over medium heat. Add the tempeh and cook until browned, about 10 minutes. Transfer the cooked tempeh to a plate and remove excess oil with paper towels.

In the same wok or skillet, add the onion and garlic, and season with salt and pepper to taste. Stir-fry over medium-high heat until the onion is soft, then add the carrots and 2 cups of water. Cover, reduce the heat to a simmer, and cook until the carrots are somewhat soft.

Add the broccoli, cover, and allow to steam until the broccoli becomes tender, 3 to 5 minutes (do not overcook). Add the reserved quinoa, tempeh, and the soy sauce. Stir to combine and serve hot.

FOREST BOWLS WITH EARTHY VEGETABLES AND TURMERIC CASHEW SAUCE

Andrea Nordby

Makes 2 servings

"The ingredients in these bowls are packed with important nutrients. Look for hemp seeds in well-stocked markets or online."

¼ cup raw unsalted macadamia nuts

¾ cup short-grain brown rice

Salt, as needed

1 clove garlic, peeled

½ teaspoon ground turmeric

1 tablespoon creamy unsalted cashew butter

Juice of ½ lemon

4 ounces enoki mushrooms, ends trimmed

1 cup vegetable broth, for steaming

Pinch of ground black pepper

6 ounces curly kale leaves, roughly chopped

10 ounces steamed red beets, cut into wedges

2 teaspoons hulled hemp seeds

4 lemon wedges

Place the macadamia nuts in a small bowl and add ⅓ cup of hot water. Set aside to soak for 3 hours or overnight.

Combine the brown rice, 1¼ cups water, and salt in a small saucepan over high heat. Bring to a boil, reduce the heat to low, cover, and cook until the rice is tender and the water is absorbed, 35 to 45 minutes.

Transfer the macadamia nuts and their soaking water into a high-speed blender. Add the garlic, turmeric, cashew butter, 1 tablespoon of the lemon juice, and a good pinch of salt. Blend until smooth, scraping down the sides of the blender as necessary. Taste the turmeric cashew sauce and add more lemon juice or salt to taste. Set aside.

Heat a large skillet over medium-high heat. Once hot, add the enoki mushrooms and a splash of vegetable broth to steam. Cook the mushrooms until tender and browned in places, about 2 to 4 minutes. Season with salt and pepper and transfer to a plate.

Immediately return the skillet to medium-high heat and add the chopped kale. Add another splash of vegetable broth to create some steam and sprinkle with salt and pepper. Cook kale until bright green and just wilted, about 2 minutes.

To serve, divide the brown rice between two large bowls and top with cooked enoki mushrooms, kale, and beets. Drizzle with turmeric cashew sauce, sprinkle with hemp seeds, and serve with lemon wedges.

BLACK BEAN TACOS

Singer, songwriter, philanthropist, and co-founder of the Meat Free Monday campaign, **Paul McCartney's** *music is loved by multiple generations the world over.*

Makes 4 servings

"Half the fun of eating tacos is making them—preparing different fillings, then piling them into the corn taco shells to your taste."

1 tablespoon olive oil

1 medium onion, or a small bunch of spring onions, chopped

One 15-ounce can black beans, drained and rinsed

2 medium tomatoes, chopped

1 teaspoon paprika

1 teaspoon ground cumin

Pinch of salt

2 teaspoons hot chili sauce (optional)

4 taco shells

1 lime, quartered

1 head Little Gem lettuce, shredded

1 ripe avocado, peeled, pitted, and sliced

Heat the oil in a large skillet over medium heat. Add the onion and cook for about 5 minutes, stirring frequently, until soft but not browned. Stir in the black beans and cook for 5 minutes. Add the chopped tomatoes, paprika, and cumin and cook, stirring until heated through. Season with salt. If you like your tacos spicy, add hot chili sauce.

To serve, warm the taco shells according to the instructions on the package and fill halfway with the bean mixture. Add a squeeze of lime and top with shredded lettuce and sliced avocado.

GREENS AND BEANS

Tracey Collins, *a long-time educator who began her career as a third grade teacher in Brooklyn, has also served as a school coordinator, assistant principal, and principal.*

Makes 2 servings

"Those with heartier appetites may want to serve this on a bed of cooked brown rice or other grain. For extra flavor, add a teaspoon of sweet chili sauce, hot sauce, or smoked balsamic vinegar, and enjoy a tasty and nutritious meal that is easy to prepare. Bonus: you can take the leftovers to work for lunch the next day."

1 cup dried red lentils

½ tablespoon ground cumin

½ tablespoon garlic powder

½ tablespoon onion powder

2 teaspoons ground turmeric

⅛ teaspoon paprika

Pinch of red pepper flakes

1 large bunch of organic kale, washed and chopped

In a saucepan, combine the lentils, cumin, garlic powder, onion powder, turmeric, paprika, and red pepper flakes. Add 4 cups of hot water and bring to a boil. Reduce the heat to a simmer with the lid ajar and cook for 20 to 25 minutes, or until desired tenderness is reached.

Steam the kale in a steamer set over a saucepan of boiling water for 5 to 7 minutes, or until desired tenderness.

Place 1 to 1½ cups of the cooked kale in a bowl. Spoon 1 cup of the cooked lentils on top of the steamed kale. Serve hot.

STOVIES

Scottish-American actor, singer, writer, producer, director, and vegan activist **Alan Cumming** *takes traditional Scottish recipes and makes them available in a plant-based version.*

Makes 8 to 10 servings

"Stovies is a Scottish dish that is traditionally made with beef drippings, but I am a vegan, so I came up with my own version. It is real peasant food—ideal for people who, like me, love to have a plateful of one thing. I much prefer a mush-style dish to something with loads of different components. Stovies are so great for parties on cold winter nights because you can just leave them on the stove and people can help themselves throughout the night as they please. You can substitute BBQ sauce, hot sauce, or mustard for all or part of the tamari and Worcestershire sauce, if you like. Basically, the trick is to make the stovies tasty and to give it a bit of a brown color. Note: If using a lot of tamari, be careful not to add too much salt."

1 to 2 tablespoons olive oil

4 cloves garlic, minced

4 large onions, chopped

8 to 10 large potatoes, well scrubbed and cut into chunks

Tamari or dark soy sauce, to taste

Vegetarian Worcestershire sauce, to taste

2 cups frozen vegan burger crumbles

Salt and ground black pepper, to taste

Heat the oil in a wok or large pot over medium heat. Add the garlic and cook until softened, about 3 minutes. Add the chopped onions to the olive oil and garlic. Cover and cook for 5 minutes, stirring occasionally. Add the potatoes and mix well.

Now comes the fun bit! Get your tamari and squirt about 20 or so squirts into the wok, then do the same with your Worcestershire sauce. Then add the vegan burger crumbles. Add enough water into the wok so that all the ingredients are just submerged. Bring to a boil, then reduce the heat to a low simmer, and continue to cook until soft, stirring occasionally, about 30 minutes, partially covered. Season with salt and pepper to taste. For a mushier texture, mash the potatoes a little with a large spoon. Cover with the lid and keep warm until serving.

SWEET POTATO–COLLARD GREEN SAAG PANEER

Raymond Jackson

Makes 4 servings

"Inspired by the traditional Indian dish made with spinach and paneer (a type of cheese), this version features ingredients from the American South with sweet potatoes standing in for the paneer and collard greens replacing the spinach."

1½ pounds sweet potatoes, peeled and cut in 1/2-inch dice

Salt and ground black pepper, to taste

Pinch of ground cinnamon

3 cups vegetable broth, divided

1 pound fresh collard greens

1 yellow onion, finely chopped

3 cloves garlic, minced

½ tablespoon finely grated fresh ginger

1 jalapeño chili, finely chopped

1½ tablespoons garam masala

1 tablespoon smoked paprika

One 14-ounce can diced tomatoes, drained

1¼ cups coconut milk

3 tablespoons tahini

Juice and zest of 1 lemon

¼ cup brown sugar

2 tablespoons chopped cilantro

4 cups cooked brown basmati rice, to serve

Preheat the oven to 350 degrees Fahrenheit. Place the diced sweet potatoes in a bowl and season liberally with salt and pepper and cinnamon. Spread the seasoned sweet potatoes in a single layer on a rimmed baking sheet lined with parchment paper or a silicone mat. If any seasoning remains in the bowl, sprinkle it on the sweet potatoes. Roast the sweet potatoes for about 30 minutes, or until they are mostly cooked, but still firm. Remove from the oven and set aside.

Bring 2 cups of the vegetable broth to a boil in a large pot. Add the collard greens and cook until they are wilted. Do not allow the greens to scorch. Remove the greens from the pot and set aside. (The broth will be almost completely evaporated.)

Return the pot to the heat. Add ¼ cup of the remaining broth and heat over medium heat. Add the onion, garlic, ginger, and jalapeño and cook, stirring frequently, until softened and browned. Stir in the garam masala and smoked paprika and cook, stirring, until fragrant. Stir in the tomatoes and remaining ¾ cup vegetable stock. Add the reserved greens and ¾ cup of the coconut milk and simmer until the greens are tender. Do not boil.

Transfer half of the greens mixture to a high-speed blender and puree to form a smooth sauce. Add the tahini, lemon juice and zest, and sugar and blend to thoroughly combine. Transfer the sauce back into the pot, add the reserved squash and remaining coconut milk if needed. Simmer until the squash is tender. Adjust the seasoning with salt and pepper if needed. Just before serving, add the cilantro. Serve over hot cooked rice.

SPICY QUINOA MEATBALLS

French-trained chef-turned-vegan **Yvonne Ardestani** *shares her recipes online in her cookbook app, Yvonne's Vegan Kitchen, and her blog,* My Eclectic Kitchen.

Makes 20 meatballs

"Fresh chilies add heat to these meatballs that can be added to your cooked marinara sauce, served on top of pasta, or enjoyed in a sandwich. They're also great smothered in a sweet and spicy barbecue sauce. Note: When working with fresh chilies, I recommend using gloves, because the hot chilies can burn your hands. If you have lime handy, rubbing your hands with lime can help alleviate any burning. And definitely don't touch your eyes when working with chilies!"

½ cup quinoa, well rinsed

1 small onion, finely chopped

1 small carrot, peeled and minced

1 large clove garlic, finely minced

2 tablespoons minced red bell pepper

2 jalapeño chilies, seeded and stemmed, finely chopped

¾ teaspoon Celtic or Himalayan sea salt

1 teaspoon dried oregano

½ teaspoon garlic powder

½ teaspoon fennel seeds

¼ teaspoon ground black pepper

⅛ teaspoon cayenne pepper

1½ cups finely chopped spinach

½ cup chopped parsley

2 tablespoons chopped fresh basil

½ cup oat flour

Preheat the oven to 400 degrees Fahrenheit.
Cook the quinoa in a saucepan with 1 cup filtered water until tender, about 15 minutes. Drain and set aside to cool.

In a large skillet over medium heat, combine the onion, carrot, garlic, bell pepper, and jalapeño and cook until the onion is translucent. (Note: You do not need any oil to sauté this mixture since the water from the onions and other veggies will seep out and will help cook the rest of the vegetables.) Add the oregano, salt, garlic powder, fennel seeds, black pepper, and cayenne pepper, cooking for about 2 minutes. Add the spinach, parsley, basil, and reserved quinoa. Stir well and cook for an additional 3 minutes.

Remove the pan from heat and add the oat flour. Stir well until everything starts to bind together and the mixture cools. If it doesn't bind together right away, add filtered water, a tablespoon at a time, up to 3 tablespoons.

Line a sheet pan with parchment paper. Using your hands, form the mixture into balls, using 2 tablespoons of the mixture per ball. (You can also use an ice cream scoop or a cookie scoop.) Arrange the balls on the sheet pan. Bake for 35 minutes or until crisp and browned. Serve immediately.

HAWAIIAN SLOPPY JACKS

Mother, vegan chef, and CEO of Jackfruit Café, **Angela Means** *is also known as the actress who portrayed Felicia in the cult-classic film* Friday. *#byefelicia*

Makes 4 servings

"We've all heard of Sloppy Joes—now we have Sloppy Jacks. Made with jackfruit, this fun take on the popular sandwich is given a Hawaiian accent with grilled pineapple. For the vegan cheese, I like to use Follow Your Heart Smoked Gouda."

2 tablespoons grapeseed oil

One 20-ounce can young green jackfruit (packed in water)

1 cup tamari sauce

½ cup pure maple syrup or agave

1½ tablespoons arrowroot powder

1 tablespoon rice vinegar

1 tablespoon onion powder

1½ teaspoons sesame oil

1½ teaspoons garlic powder

½ teaspoon sea salt

½ teaspoon ground black pepper

⅛ teaspoon powdered ginger

4 pineapple rings

4 red onion ring slices

4 vegan brioche buns or other burger rolls

8 vegan cheese slices

12 slices pickled jalapeño

1 cup alfalfa spouts

Heat 1½ tablespoons of the grapeseed oil in a large cast-iron skillet over medium heat. Add the jackfruit and cook, stirring occasionally until tender, about 45 minutes. Add a splash of water to prevent it from scorching, as needed. Use two forks to shred the jackfruit while cooking. Continue to shred and stir well as the jackfruit cooks. Do not let it scorch.

Combine the tamari, maple syrup, arrowroot powder, rice vinegar, onion powder, sesame oil, garlic powder, sea salt, ground black pepper, and ginger in a saucepan. Cook at a simmer, stirring occasionally until hot and thickened. If the sauce becomes too thick, stir in up to ½ cup boiling water, a little at a time, as needed. Pour the sauce over the cooked jackfruit and simmer 10 minutes, stirring constantly.

Heat the remaining ½ tablespoon of grapeseed oil in a large skillet over medium-high heat. Add the pineapple and grill to your preference. Remove the pineapple rings from the skillet and set aside. Add the onion ring slices to the skillet and grill to your preference.

To assemble sandwiches, arrange one bun open on a plate. Place 1 slice of vegan cheese on the bun, then top with a large spoonful of the prepared jackfruit, followed by 1 pineapple ring, 1 onion ring, a second cheese slice, 3 pickled jalapeño slices, and ¼ cup sprouts. Repeat with the remaining ingredients to make four sandwiches and serve immediately.

GRITS AND GREENS

Robin Robertson

Makes 4 servings

"Nutritional yeast gives these grits a slightly cheesy flavor without the cheese, but you can stir in up to ½ cup of shredded vegan cheddar, if you like, for even more cheesy goodness. For another delicious addition, cook up some chopped vegan bacon and stir it into the grits or sprinkle it on top of the greens when ready to serve."

1 cup grits	½ cup minced onion
2 tablespoons nutritional yeast	3 cloves garlic, minced
2 scallions, finely minced	1 teaspoon liquid smoke
2 teaspoons vegan butter	½ teaspoon smoked paprika
Salt and ground black pepper, to taste	4 cups chopped collard greens
1 tablespoon olive oil	½ cup vegetable broth

Cook the grits according to package directions. (Instant grits should take about 5 minutes.) Stir in the nutritional yeast, scallions, vegan butter, and salt and pepper to taste. Keep warm.

While the grits are cooking, heat the oil in a large skillet over medium heat. Add the onion and garlic and cook 5 minutes to soften. Sprinkle on the liquid smoke and smoked paprika, tossing to coat. Add the greens and broth, and season with salt and pepper to taste. Cook, stirring, until the greens are tender, 5 to 10 minutes. Taste and adjust the seasonings if needed.

To serve, spoon the grits onto plates or shallow bowls and top with the greens.

PASTA WITH CHARRED TOMATOES AND WHITE WINE SAUCE

Leslie Durso *is a vegan chef and wellness expert who consults for resorts and restaurants around the world while also working as the vegan chef at the Four Seasons, Punta Mita, Mexico.*

Makes 4 servings

"Charring is the process of slightly roasting tomatoes so they get a brown, slightly burned skin. As with all heat applications, this allows for more sugars to develop, and the charred skin adds a slightly smoky flavor component while reducing the water content of the tomatoes. Grape or cherry tomatoes are ideal for this process, as they are small and have a large amount of surface area."

¼ cup extra-virgin olive oil	1 teaspoon sea salt
32 ounces grape tomatoes	¼ teaspoon ground black pepper
4 tablespoons chopped garlic	1 pound of your favorite pasta
One 750-milliliter bottle Pinot Grigio	8 to 10 fresh basil leaves, chopped

Put a pot of salted water on to boil for the pasta.

Heat the oil in a large skillet over medium-high heat. Add the tomatoes and cook, allowing them to sizzle and begin to pop, about 5 minutes. Once they are popping and golden on the bottom, begin to swirl your pan around carefully as to not break the tomatoes. Cook another 2 minutes. Add the garlic and carefully pour in the wine until the tomatoes are almost covered in the wine. As the wine evaporates and cooks down, continue to add wine until you've used the whole bottle. Season the sauce with salt and pepper. Keep warm.

When the pasta water comes to a boil, add the pasta and cook until the pasta is just tender, about 10 minutes. Drain the pasta, then toss the pasta in the reserved tomato sauce. Top with freshly chopped basil and serve hot.

AFRICAN GREENS MÉLANGE

CC Péan

Makes 4 servings

"This healthier take on a soul-food tradition can be served as a side dish or, as shown here, it can become a hearty main dish with the optional addition of cooked beans and served on a bed of cooked rice. Note: If you are adding the optional Scotch bonnet chili, be sure to use gloves when handling it."

2 tablespoons coconut oil

1 yellow onion, thinly sliced

4 cloves garlic, minced

1 red bell pepper, thinly sliced

1 yellow bell pepper, thinly sliced

1 celery stalk, thinly sliced

½ Scotch bonnet chili, seeded and thinly sliced (optional)

2 bunches lacinato or dinosaur kale, rolled and thinly sliced

1 bunch collard greens, rolled and thinly sliced

1 teaspoon smoked paprika

⅓ cup vegetable broth

Pinch of salt

One 15-ounce can black-eyed peas, drained and rinsed (optional)

4 cups cooked brown rice, to serve (optional)

Heat the oil in a large pot over medium-high heat. Add the onion and cook until it is translucent, stirring occasionally. Add the garlic, bell peppers, celery, and Scotch bonnet chili, if using. Cook for about 2 minutes.

Add the greens and smoked paprika, stirring until the greens begin to wilt and all the ingredients are evenly distributed. Add the vegetable broth and cover the pot. Let the vegetables steam for about 5 minutes, stirring occasionally to prevent sticking. Season with salt to taste. Stir in the black-eyed peas, if using, and heat for a minute or two to heat through. Serve hot over cooked brown rice, if desired.

B.Y. BURGERS

Bryant Jennings *is an American heavyweight boxer from Philadelphia, Pennsylvania, who turned pro in February 2010 and went on to score 19 straight wins. He went totally vegan in 2015.*

Makes 8 servings

"Make the burger mixture ahead of when you need them. If you don't plan to cook all the burgers at once, you can freeze the rest until needed—just make sure to wrap them individually or separate them with a small square of waxed paper so they don't stick together in the freezer."

⅓ cup quinoa, rinsed and drained

One 15-ounce can black beans, drained and rinsed

One 15-ounce can chickpeas, drained and rinsed

1 tablespoon chia seeds

1 red bell pepper, finely chopped

¼ cup candied walnuts, roughly chopped

½ cup breadcrumbs

½ cup tomato paste

1 teaspoon onion powder

1 teaspoon garlic powder

1 teaspoon salt

½ teaspoon paprika

1 to 2 tablespoons chopped fresh parsley

1 tablespoon olive oil

8 vegan brioche buns, lightly toasted

Optional toppings: lettuce leaves, tomato slices, onion slices, pickle chips, mustard, relish

Cook the quinoa according to the package directions, about 15 minutes. Drain off any excess water and set aside to cool.

In a large mixing bowl, combine the black beans and chickpeas. Add the chia seeds and stir to combine.

Stir in the cooked quinoa, bell pepper, walnuts, breadcrumbs, tomato paste, onion powder, garlic powder, salt, paprika, and parsley. Mix well to combine, then use a potato masher to mash the mixture until all the ingredients hold together well. Cover the mixture and refrigerate for at least 20 minutes or overnight.

With clean hands, scoop a small handful of the mixture and press it into a ball, then use your hands to flatten it into a patty, and place on a clean work surface. Repeat with the remaining burgers. The burgers are now ready to cook.

Heat the olive oil in a nonstick skillet over medium heat. Add the burgers and cook for 3 to 5 minutes, then flip the burgers and cook for another 3 to 5 minutes, or until cooked and golden brown.

Serve on burger buns with your favorite toppings.

DESSERTS

THREE-INGREDIENT ICE CREAM

For the past three decades, **Eric Adams** *has served the residents of Brooklyn as borough president, state senator, police officer, and coalition builder. In November of 2017, he was reelected for a second term to represent Brooklyn as borough president. He is running for mayor of New York in 2021.*

Makes 1 to 2 servings

"There's nothing wrong with occasionally enjoying a healthy, plant-based dessert. The key is keeping the portions small. Here, alongside the pure deliciousness, come the health benefits of bananas, cacao powder, and cacao nibs (filled with antioxidants, magnesium, iron, fiber, protein, and healthy fats). Sometimes I like to sprinkle cacao nibs in other desserts as well; they make everything taste chocolatey good."

3 medium bananas, peeled, sliced, and frozen for a few hours or overnight

1 tablespoon cacao powder

2 to 4 tablespoons cacao nibs or nuts of your choice (optional)

Combine all the ingredients in a food processor. Process until the texture changes from crumbly to creamy. Transfer to a bowl and serve right away or place the bowl in the freezer for an hour or so for a firmer texture.

BASMATI RICE PUDDING

Originally from Guyana, **Dr. Fiona B. Lewis,** *who grew up in the Bronx, New York, is a doctor of public health, registered dietician, and plant-based chef.*

Makes 4 servings

"Rice is a celebrated staple in many cultures. It is one of the most versatile culinary ingredients. It can be used to make both savory and sweet dishes. This recipe is inspired by the rice porridge my mother and grandmother made for breakfast. They didn't have an ingredient as sophisticated as basmati rice; white rice was the main ingredient for Guyanese-style rice porridge. To add extra layers of flavor, I replaced the traditional nutmeg with cardamom and white rice with basmati brown rice. This aromatic whole grain is more nutrient dense because the germ and the endosperm of the rice grain have not been removed. The interesting flavors in this rice pudding are enhanced when it is topped with some orange zest."

1½ teaspoons cardamom seeds	½ teaspoon sea salt
¾ cup brown basmati rice	1 teaspoon vanilla extract
1 cup light coconut milk	Zest from 1 orange (optional)
2½ cups unsweetened nondairy milk, such as almond or soy milk	Optional toppings: chopped fresh fruit, toasted coconut, toasted almond slivers, or chopped nuts
⅓ cup maple syrup	

Toast the cardamom seeds in a small pan over medium heat for 2 to 3 minutes. Remove from the heat. Cool for 5 minutes then grind in a spice grinder and set aside.

Rinse the rice and place it in a nonstick pot. Stir the rice with a spoon over medium heat until it is dry. Add the ground cardamom, coconut milk, nondairy milk, ⅔ cup water, maple syrup, salt, and vanilla and bring it to a boil. Simmer on low to medium heat with the pot half-covered for 40 to 50 minutes. Check to make sure rice grains are soft and creamy before removing the pot from the heat. Add ¼ cup water if the pudding is too thick or the rice is not fully cooked. Be sure to taste the pudding and adjust the flavor if extra water is added. Top with the orange zest and optional toppings, if using. Serve warm or cold.

NO-BAKE SWEET POTATO BARS WITH RAW GINGERBREAD CRUST

Jenné Claiborne

Makes 6 to 8 servings

"This recipe is adapted from a no-bake pumpkin bar recipe on *The Kitchn* blog. Pumpkin can be used in place of the sweet potato if that's what you've got."

1 cup almonds	Pinch of sea salt
½ cup shredded unsweetened coconut	½ cup coconut oil
	1½ cups sweet potato puree
1½ cups Medjool dates, pitted	⅓ cup maple syrup
1 tablespoon molasses	1 teaspoon freshly squeezed
½-inch piece ginger, minced	lemon juice
2½ teaspoons ground cinnamon	1 teaspoon vanilla extract
¼ teaspoon ground nutmeg	¼ teaspoon salt
½ teaspoon ground cloves, divided	¾ teaspoon ground cardamom
	¾ teaspoon ground ginger
¼ teaspoon cayenne pepper	2 tablespoons coconut flour
Pinch of ground black pepper	

Line an 8 x 8-inch baking pan with parchment paper.

Place the almonds, coconut, dates, molasses, ginger, 1 teaspoon cinnamon, nutmeg, ¼ teaspoon ground cloves, cayenne, black pepper, sea salt, and 1 tablespoon coconut oil in a food processor and blend until well combined. Remove the lid and gather some of the mixture into your hand, squeezing it to form a tight ball in your palm. If the crust crumbles and doesn't stick, you'll need to blend it some more or add another date.

Transfer the crust mixture into the prepared baking pan and press it firmly to the bottom to create a tight crust. Set aside.

Place the sweet potato puree, maple syrup, remaining coconut oil, lemon juice, vanilla, salt, 1½ teaspoons cinnamon, cardamom, ground ginger, remaining ground cloves, pinch of black pepper, and coconut flour in a food processor and blend until smooth. Taste, and add more maple syrup if necessary. Spoon the filling into the crust and smooth down with the back of a large spoon or rubber spatula.

Place the pan in the refrigerator for about 6 hours or overnight to allow it to set. Grasp the sides of the parchment paper to pull the dessert out of the pan. Place it on a cutting board and cut it into bars. Any uneaten bars can be stored in the refrigerator for up to a week.

EASY CHOCOLATE TRUFFLES

Robin Robertson

Makes 10 to 12 truffles

"Dates provide the sweetness in these chocolatey truffles that only taste decadent."

½ cup pitted dates	¼ cup almond butter
⅓ cup unsweetened cocoa powder	⅓ cup toasted slivered almonds, finely ground (optional)

Soak the pitted dates in warm water for at least 30 minutes. Drain the dates well and transfer to a food processor. Process until finely minced. Add the cocoa and almond butter and process until well combined. The mixture should hold together when pinched. If the mixture is too loose, blend in a little more cocoa powder. If it is too dry, blend in a few teaspoons of water, 1 teaspoon at a time.

Line a plate with plastic film wrap. Use your hands to shape the mixture into 1-inch balls and set on the plate. If coating the truffles in almonds, place the ground almonds in a shallow bowl. Roll the truffles in the ground almonds, pressing to coat. Arrange the truffles on a plate and refrigerate for at least 1 hour, or until firm.

CHEWY PEANUT BUTTER COOKIES

Charity Morgan

Makes 6 to 8 servings

"The simplest things are sometimes the best, like these 3-ingredient, vegan, gluten-free chewy peanut butter cookies. I like to devour these with a cold glass of almond milk."

1 cup peanut butter

1 cup maple syrup

1 cup gluten-free flour

1 teaspoon vanilla extract (optional)

Preheat the oven to 350 degrees Fahrenheit. Line a baking sheet with a silicone mat or a sheet of parchment paper. Set aside.

Combine all the ingredients in a bowl and mix well, using a rubber spatula. Roll the mixture into 1-inch balls and arrange them on the prepared baking sheet. Use a fork to press into the balls to flatten them slightly. Bake for 15 to 20 minutes, or until golden brown.

FRUIT PIZZA

Donna Green-Goodman

Makes 6 to 8 servings

"If you're short on time and don't want to make the crust, you can use a store-bought pie crust, such as Bob's Red Mill Gluten Free Pie Crust."

1 cup walnut pieces

1 cup cashew pieces

¾ cup slivered almonds

1 cup pitted dates

4 ounces nondairy cream cheese

3 ounces nondairy whipped cream

6 ounces nondairy sour cream

One 5-ounce container nondairy vanilla yogurt

⅓ cup sliced strawberries

⅓ cup sliced blueberries

⅓ cup sliced blackberries

½ cup diced pineapple

½ cup sliced kiwi

To make the pie crust, combine the walnuts, cashews, and almonds in a food processor and process until coarsely ground. Add the dates and process until they are finely chopped and incorporated into the nuts. The mixture should come together like a dough. (If it is too dry to hold together, add 1 teaspoon of water.)

Line a pizza pan with parchment paper. Transfer the crust mixture to the prepared pizza pan and spread it out thinly and evenly with damp fingers, shaping it into a round-bottom crust.

Whisk together the cream cheese, whipped cream, sour cream, and yogurt until light and fluffy. Spread on top of the crust.

Arrange the berries, pineapple, and kiwi on top of the pie. Refrigerate the fruit pizza until well chilled, at least 1 hour. Serve.

ENDNOTES

Introduction

1. "Diabetes: Tackle Diabetes with a Plant-Based Diet," Physicians Committee for Responsible Medicine, accessed October 12, 2019, https://www.pcrm.org/health-topics/diabetes.

Chapter 1

1. "Heart Disease," Centers for Disease Control and Prevention, accessed September 30, 2019, https://www.cdc.gov/heartdisease/about.htm.

2. "Statistics about Diabetes," American Diabetes Association, https://www.diabetes.org/resources/statistics/statistics-about-diabetes.

3. Andrew Gerald Shaper, "Serum-Cholesterol, Diet, and Coronary Heart-Disease in Africans and Asians in Uganda: 1959," *International Journal of Epidemiology* 41, no. 5 (October 2012): 1221–1225.

4. "Nathan Pritikin, Founder," Pritikin Longevity Center, accessed October 2, 2019, https://www.pritikin.com/home-the-basics/about-pritikin/38-nathan-pritikin.html.

5. Michael Greger, *How Not to Die: Discover the Foods Scientifically Proven to Prevent and Reverse Disease* (New York: Flatiron Books, 2015), ix.

6. Greger, *How Not to Die*, x.

7. Joe Conason, "Bill Clinton Explains Why He Became a Vegan," *AARP The Magazine,* August/September 2013, https://www.aarp.org/health/healthy-living/info-08-2013/bill-clinton-vegan.html.

8. Gabrielle Turner-McGrievy et al., "The Nutritious Eating with Soul (NEW Soul) Study: Study Design and Methods of a Two-Year Randomized Trial Comparing Culturally Adapted Soul Food Vegan vs. Omnivorous Diets Among African American Adults at Risk for Heart Disease," *Contemporary Clinical Trials* 88, (January 2020), doi: 10.1016/j.cct.2019.105897.

9. "The Heart Attack Gender Gap," Harvard Health Publishing, published April 2016, https://www.health.harvard.edu/heart-health/the-heart-attack-gender-gap.

10. "Halt Heart Disease with a Plant-Based, Oil-Free Diet," Harvard Health Publishing, published September 2014, https://www.health.harvard.edu/heart-disease-overview/halt-heart-disease-with-a-plant-based-oil-free-diet-.

11. Serena Tonstad et al., "Vegetarian Diets and Incidence of Diabetes in the Adventist Health Study-2," *Nutrition, Metabolism & Cardiovascular Diseases* 23, no. 4 (April 2013): 292–299.

12. "Tackle Diabetes," Physicians Committee for Responsible Medicine.

13. "How Common Is Breast Cancer?" American Cancer Society, accessed March 16, 2020, https://www.cancer.org/cancer/breast-cancer/about/how-common-is-breast-cancer.html.

14. Carol Desantis et al., "Breast Cancer Statistics, 2019," *CA: A Cancer Journal for Physicians* 69, no. 6 (October 2019): 438–451.

15. Rowan T. Chlebowski et al, "Low-Fat Dietary Pattern and Long-Term Breast Cancer Incidence and Mortality: The Women's Health Initiative Randomized Clinical Trial," Abstract presented at the 2019 American Society of Clinical Oncology annual meeting, Chicago, May 31–June 4, 2019.

16. Faye Taylor et al., "Meat Consumption and Risk of Breast Cancer in the UK Women's Cohort Study," *British Journal of Cancer* 96, no. 7 (April 2007): 1139–1146.

17. Katherine Zeratsky, "Will Eating Soy Increase My Risk of Breast Cancer?," Mayo Clinic, accessed September 30, 2019, https://www.mayoclinic.org/healthy-lifestyle/nutrition-and-healthy-eating/expert-answers/soy-breast-cancer-risk/faq-20120377.

18. "Soy Linked to Breast Cancer Survival," Physicians Committee for Responsible Medicine, published March 6, 2017, https://www.pcrm.org/news/health-nutrition/soy-linked-breast-cancer-survival.

19. "Key Statistics for Prostate Cancer," American Cancer Society, accessed March 16, 2020, https://www.cancer.org/cancer/prostate-cancer/about/key-statistics.html.

20. "African Americans and Prostate Cancer," Zero: The End of Prostate Cancer, accessed March 16, 2020, https://zerocancer.org/learn/about-prostate-cancer/risks/african-americans-prostate-cancer/.

21. Sarah Lewis, "Milk and Prostate Cancer—How Are They Linked?," World Cancer Research Fund International, published May 8, 2017, https://www.wcrf.org/int/blog/articles/2017/05/milk-and-prostate-cancer-how-are-they-linked.

22. Greger, *How Not to Die*, 214.

23. "Cancer: Reducing Cancer Risk with a Plant-Based Diet," Physicians Committee for Responsible Medicine, accessed October 21, 2019, https://www.pcrm.org/health-topics/cancer.

24. Farhad Islami et al., "Proportion and Number of Cancer Cases and Deaths Attributable to Potentially Modifiable Risk Factors in the United States," *CA: A Cancer Journal for Clinicians* 68, no. 1 (January 2018): 31–54.

25. "2018 Alzheimer's Disease Facts and Figures," Alzheimer's Association, accessed March 16, 2020, https://www.alz.org/aaic/_downloads/aaic-facts-and-figures -fact-sheet-2018.pdf.

26. Greger, *How Not to Die*, 54.

27. Paul Giem et al., "The Incidence of Dementia and Intake of Animal Products: Preliminary Findings from the Adventist Health Study," *Neuroepidemiology* 12, no. 1 (May 1993): 28–36.

28. "Researchers Say Most Alzheimer's Disease Cases Are Preventable—Find Out How," Blue Zones, accessed Dec. 2, 2019, https://www.bluezones.com/2017/09 /researchers-say-alzheimers-disease-cases-preventable-find/.

29. L.J. Gambone, "Loma Linda Doctors Say You Can Prevent or Turn Around Alzheimer's Disease," *Daily Press,* updated May 15, 2018, https://www .vvdailypress.com/news/20180509/loma-linda-doctors-say-you-can-prevent -or-turn-around-alzheimers-disease.

30. Amanda Baltazar, "Do Vegan or Vegetarian Diets Help Reduce Arthritis Inflammation?," Arthritis Foundation, accessed October 12, 2019, https:// www.arthritis.org/living-with-arthritis/arthritis-diet/anti-inflammatory /vegan-and-vegetarian-diets.php.

31. Feng Wang et al., "Erectile Dysfunction and Fruit/Vegetable Consumption Among Diabetic Canadian Men," *Urology* 82, no. 6 (December 2013): 1330– 1335.

32. Jemima Webber, "Going Vegan Is Better Than Viagra, Says James Cameron," *LIVEKINDLY,* published April 8, 2019, https://www.livekindly.co/james -cameron-believes-veganism-can-put-viagra-out-of-business/.

33. "Skin Conditions by the Numbers," American Academy of Dermatology, accessed March 16, 2020, https://www.aad.org/media/stats-numbers.

34. Loren Cordain et al., "Acne Vulgaris: A Disease of Western Civilization," *Archives of Dermatology* 138, no. 12 (December 2002): 1584–1590.

35. Ye Li et al., "Dietary Patterns and Depression Risk: A Meta-Analysis," *Psychiatry Research* 253 (July 2017): 373–382.

Chapter 2

1. Adrian Miller, *Soul Food: The Surprising Story of an American Cuisine, One Plate at a Time* (Chapel Hill: University of North Carolina Press, 2013) Kindle edition, chap. 6.

2. Luke Johnson, "Pat Robertson on Mac and Cheese: 'Is That a Black Thing?'" *Huffington Post,* updated December 6, 2017, https://www.huffpost.com/entry /pat-robertson-mac-and-cheese-black-thing_n_1110659.

3. Kastalia Medrano, "Kitchen of Thomas Jefferson's Slave, Who Brought Mac and Cheese to America, Discovered at Monticello Plantation," *Newsweek,* published January 11, 2018, https://www.newsweek.com/kitchen-thomas-jeffersons -slave-chef-james-hemings-macaroni-and-cheese-america-777425.

4. Miller, *Soul Food,* chap. 8.

5. "What Is Soul Food?" *Delish,* published February 15, 2019, https://www.delish
.com/food-news/a26356466/what-is-soul-food/.

6. Alex Park, "How the Fast-Food Industry Courted African American Customers,"
Washington Post, published June 11, 2018, https://www.washingtonpost.com
/news/made-by-history/wp/2018/06/11/the-origins-of-fast-foods-enduring
-popularity-with-african-americans/.

7. Park, "How the Fast-Food Industry Courted African American Customers,"
Washington Post.

8. Roberto Ferdman, "The Disturbing Ways That Fast Food Chains
Disproportionately Target Black Kids," *Washington Post,* published November
12, 2014, https://www.washingtonpost.com/news/wonk/wp/2014/11/12/the
-disturbing-ways-that-fast-food-chains-disproportionately-target-black-kids/.

9. "Cancer Facts & Figures for African Americans 2019–2021," American Cancer
Society, https://www.cancer.org/content/dam/cancer-org/research/cancer
-facts-and-statistics/cancer-facts-and-figures-for-african-americans/cancer
-facts-and-figures-for-african-americans-2019-2021.pdf.

10. Kathleen Hall, "Why Are African-Americans at Greater Risk for Colorectal
Cancer?," *U.S. News & World Report,* published July 5, 2017, https://health
.usnews.com/health-care/patient-advice/articles/2017-07-05/why-are
-african-americans-at-greater-risk-for-colorectal-cancer.

11. Miller, *Soul Food,* chap. 9.

12. Miller, *Soul Food,* chap. 2.

13. Sam Collins, "What Happened When Scientists Put African Americans on an
African Diet and Africans on an American Diet," *Think Progress,* published
May 15, 2015, https://thinkprogress.org/what-happened-when-scientists
-put-african-americans-on-an-african-diet-and-africans-on-an-american
-5b5c5aec6e1e/.

14. Ibram Kendi, "The Greatest White Privilege Is Life Itself," *The Atlantic,*
published October 24, 2019, https://www.theatlantic.com/ideas
/archive/2019/10/too-short-lives-black-men/600628/.

15. Linda Villarosa, "Myths about Physical Racial Differences Were Used to Justify
Slavery—and Are Still Believed by Doctors Today," *New York Times Magazine,*
published August 14, 2019, https://www.nytimes.com/interactive/2019/08/14
/magazine/racial-differences-doctors.html.

16. Katrina Armstrong et al., "Racial/Ethnic Differences in Physician Distrust in
the United States," *American Journal of Public Health* 97, no. 7 (July 2007):
1283–1289.

Chapter 3

1. "Cutting Red Meat for a Longer Life," Harvard Health Publishing, published June 2012, https://www.health.harvard.edu/staying-healthy/cutting-red-meat-for-a-longer-life.

2. Margaret Murphy et al., "Whole Beetroot Consumption Acutely Improves Running Performance," *Journal of the Academy of Nutrition and Dietetics* 112, no. 4 (April 2012): 548–552.

3. Neal Barnard, *21-Day Weight Loss Kickstart: Boost Metabolism, Lower Cholesterol, and Dramatically Improve Your Health* (New York: Grand Central, 2011), Kindle edition, chap. 5.

INDEX

NOTE: Page references in *italics* following names of people refer to recipes created by that person.

ACKNOWLEDGMENTS

Thank you to my partner in life and in health, Tracey Collins. We embarked on this plant-based adventure together, and she was there for me every step of the way. I cannot wait to see where our journey brings us next.

I would like to thank my strategist and friend, Rachel Atcheson, whose infectious passion for plant-based eating helped convince me to write this book. She worked tirelessly alongside me at Borough Hall, and in her very limited free time, she worked tirelessly on this book. It would never have been possible without her wisdom and energy, and I am forever grateful.

Dr. Caldwell Esselstyn invited me to his seminar in Cleveland and patiently explained to me how and why I needed to change my diet. His work has saved countless lives, including my own.

Dr. Michael Greger is the most devoted champion for plant-based eating on the face of the planet. He does more work at his treadmill desk before 9 A.M. than most of us do in a month. His website, nutritionfacts.org, remains a bible for me and millions of others around the world.

When my office galvanized the launch of a plant-based nutrition program in New York City's municipal hospital system, Dr. Michelle McMacken enthusiastically agreed to take the lead. Under her stewardship, the Plant-Based Lifestyle Medicine Program at NYC Health + Hospitals/Bellevue has garnered great enthusiasm among physicians and patients alike and helped many New Yorkers lose weight, reverse type 2 diabetes, and improve their high blood pressure, high cholesterol, heart disease, and other chronic ailments. Her time and effort helped make this book possible, but more important, she is saving lives across our city.

I am indebted to my dear friends Cliff Hollingsworth and Jacqui Williams. Witnessing your journeys to health has inspired me to spread the message of plant-based eating to all New Yorkers. I would also like to thank those who generously donated their time to be interviewed for this book, including Dr. Neal Barnard, Dr. Columbus Batiste, Dr. Judy Brangman, Marilyn Jackson, Ingrid Lewis-Martin, Rev. Fred Lucas, Dr. Milton Mills, Dr. Baxter Montgomery, Dr. Bobby Price, Marline Thomas, Dr. Brie Turner, and Rev. Al Sharpton. Finally, I am immensely grateful to Dr. Kim Williams, who wrote the wonderful foreword to this book.

This book would not have been complete without healthy and delicious recipes! Thank you to the talented chefs who generously shared their creations: Dorothy Adams, Queen Afua, Yvonne Ardestani, Dotsie Bausch, Marco Borges, Gregory Brown, Suzy Amis Cameron, Jenné Claiborne, Tracey Collins, Alan Cumming, Nina Curtis, Leslie Durso, Caldwell Esselstyn, Rip Esselstyn, Donna Green-Goodman, Dr. Michael Greger, Ayinde Howell, Raymond Jackson, B.Y. Jennings, Dr. Fiona B. Lewis, John Lewis, Taymer Mason, Paul McCartney, Dr. Michelle McMacken, Angela Means, Zakiyaa Michèl, Moby, Charity Morgan, Andrea Nordby, CC Péan, Robin Robertson, Megan Sadd, Chad Sarno and Derek Sarno, Del Sroufe, Darshana Thacker, and Dominick Thompson.

Thank you to my literary agents, Richard Pine and Eliza Rothstein. Richard, Eliza, and the rest of the Inkwell team helped shape this book from the beginning and patiently guided me through the process of finding a publisher. And that publisher turned out to be the wonderful folks at Hay House, whose kind words and strong vision immediately won me over. Six months later the manuscript was deftly edited by Sally Mason-Swaab, whose constructive feedback and shrewd eye brought my writing to a new level. I would also like to thank the rest of the Hay House team, including Adaobi Tulton, Marlene Robinson, Lindsay McGinty, and Sierra Hernandez.

A big thank you to Tommy Thomas and Brianna Suggs for creating such a beautiful book cover, and to the brilliant Rocco and Sabina Scazzariello, who made me look like an Iron Chef!

Acknowledgments

My co-writers Gene Stone and Nicholas Bromley helped coax my thoughts into words and then onto the page. They cheerfully adapted to my crazy schedule and always remained the consummate professionals. Chef extraordinaire Robin Robertson edited the recipes in this book and ensured each were healthy, straightforward, and delicious.

Thank you to the people of Brooklyn, who did me the distinct honor of letting me serve them as a police officer, a state senator, and as borough president. Brooklyn will forever be my home, and it is truly the most special place on earth.

Finally, thank you to my mother, Dorothy Adams. Watching her heal her body gave me the strength to help other New Yorkers heal theirs. I wake up every morning and go to bed every night determined to make her proud.

ABOUT THE AUTHOR

For the past three decades, Eric Adams has served the residents of Brooklyn as borough president, state senator, police officer, and coalition builder. In November of 2017, he was reelected for a second term to represent Brooklyn as borough president. Born in Brownsville and educated in the city's public school system, he is committed to ensuring Brooklyn's bright future by helping each and every Brooklynite reach his or her full potential.

We hope you enjoyed this Hay House book. If you'd like to receive our online catalog featuring additional information on Hay House books and products, or if you'd like to find out more about the Hay Foundation, please contact:

Hay House, Inc., P.O. Box 5100, Carlsbad, CA 92018-5100
(760) 431-7695 or (800) 654-5126
(760) 431-6948 (fax) or (800) 650-5115 (fax)
www.hayhouse.com® • www.hayfoundation.org

———

Published in Australia by: Hay House Australia Pty. Ltd.,
18/36 Ralph St., Alexandria NSW 2015
Phone: 612-9669-4299 • *Fax:* 612-9669-4144
www.hayhouse.com.au

Published in the United Kingdom by: Hay House UK, Ltd.,
The Sixth Floor, Watson House, 54 Baker Street, London W1U 7BU
Phone: +44 (0)20 3927 7290 • *Fax:* +44 (0)20 3927 7291
www.hayhouse.co.uk

Published in India by: Hay House Publishers India,
Muskaan Complex, Plot No. 3, B-2, Vasant Kunj, New Delhi 110 070
Phone: 91-11-4176-1620 • *Fax:* 91-11-4176-1630
www.hayhouse.co.in

———

Access New Knowledge.
Anytime. Anywhere.

Learn and evolve at your own pace
with the world's leading experts.

www.hayhouseU.com